THE HEALTHY BENEFITS OF SIRT FOOD DIET

ACTIVATE YOUR SKINNY GENE AND BOOST METABOLISM TO EASILY BURN FAT AND LOSE WEIGHT FAST, WHILE EATING THE FOODS YOU LOVE. INCLUDING MANY DELICIOUS RECIPES.

GRACE RICHARDSON

© Copyright 2020 - All rights reserved.

Table Of Contents

Introduction **6**

Chapter 1: A Scientific Approach To Diet And Health **8**

Chapter 2: Empirical Study **14**

Chapter 3: Advantages Of Sirt Food Diet **18**

Chapter 4: Sirtfood Around The World **22**

Chapter 5: Sirt Vs Keto Diet: A Comparison **28**

Chapter 6: Top 20 Sirt Food **34**

Chapter 7: Benefit Effects..**42**

Chapter 8: Weight Loss **46**

Chapter 9: Sirtfood Diet And Workout...**50**

Chapter 10: The Right Mindset To Lose Weight **54**

Chapter 11: Step By Step Sirtfood Diet..**58**

Chapter 12: Post Diet **68**

Chapter 13: Breakfast Recipes **72**

Chapter 14: Lunch Recipes...**78**

Chapter 15: Snack Recipes **86**

Chapter 16: Dinner Recipes..**92**

Chapter 17: Dessert Recipes...**100**

Conclusion **106**

Introduction

The Sirtfood Diet is a new diet that was designed in the UK, created by celebrity nutritionists, Aidan Goggins and Glen Matten, and published in a recipe book in 2016. Designed to allow for you to eat certain foods that will enable you to trigger your skinny gene, the diet is designed to help people rapidly shed the pounds without the same consequences that are commonly seen in other fad diets. Some diets require you to starve yourself and wind up, causing loss of muscle along with the fat. Others need you to give up on foods that you enjoy, making them so restrictive that they are difficult for most people to keep up with. However, the Sirtfood Diet encourages you to focus on sirtuin-rich foods that can be combined into meals that are delicious and satisfying. How does chicken curry sound? You can consume it on the Sirtfood Diet. What about a nice turmeric salmon? That is also a meal that you can enjoy. You can even enjoy blueberry pancakes for breakfast on this diet as well.

The Sirtfood Diet, as has been mentioned, is a diet in which you can provide yourself with higher than normal levels of sirtuin-rich foods so that you can use those sirtuins to activate the proteins within your body to teach it to be able to spur its weight loss. When Goggins and Matten got together to study sirtfoods, they decided that they would experiment with them; they ultimately designed a diet that served to increase and maximize sirtfood intake while also encouraging mild calorie restrictions. Together, they found that on average, participants who took this challenge consumed the sirtuin-rich foods, and restricted their calories to between 1000-1500kCal per day were able to see dramatic weight loss, even without any increase in exercising or activity. On average, during that first week, the members lost 7 pounds without doing much else other than changing their diet. Does that sound promising to you?

Even better, these people reported that they were able to gain muscle rather than losing it—something that is practically unheard of in the diet world. Typically, weight loss comes with muscle loss as well, but these individuals built it. They also reported that they were happier and healthier in general—their mental health and general wellbeing increased as well.

Overall, there are some pretty compelling reasons to start considering the Sirtfood Diet—if you want to lose weight, gain muscle, and be healthier, and this is a great way to be able to do this. It will take diligence and dedication, but if you can make sure that you commit to this process, you, too, can reap these benefits. You can begin to be a healthier individual, inside and out.

Now, you may be wondering if the Sirtfood Diet is right for you. It may be—if you are healthy otherwise and you know that you can tolerate those calorie restrictions, then this diet will probably be just fine for you. Do you have the dedication and the willpower to follow it? There is nothing worse for your weight-loss attempts than failing to see progress or failing to stick to it, so if you feel like you cannot make this diet work for you, you may not be in the right place.

Remember, even if you do not or cannot follow through with the restrictions, there is still a great benefit to adding the sirtuin-rich foods to your diet. As we will address shortly, many of the foods that you can get in that are rich in sirtuins are already highly nutritious and recognized as dietary powerhouses. There is no doubt about it—the foods that you will consume during this diet are right for you. They are very healthy, and they should be included in your diet whether you want to follow the Sirtfood Diet or not.

CHAPTER 1:

A Scientific Approach to Diet and Health

The term 'sirtfood' refers to a natural or slightly processed food item that contains a set of special chemicals known as polyphenols. The polyphenols in the sirtfoods have the ability to lead to the activation of a set of genes in the body known as 'sirtuins.' The sirtuins are also known as skinny genes, and when they are activated, they are able to trigger weight loss in a person. That's basically how sirtfoods work, in a nutshell.

Slim Gene or Sirtuins

All foods certified as sirtfood have all been extensively analyzed to understand their compositions and their effects on the body. One thing that has been found in all sirtfoods is that they contain a couple of compounds known collectively as polyphenols. The first sirtfood was analyzed in the 20th century, and it was the skin of red grapes used in making red wine. During the analysis of these skins, it was found out that these skins contained a polyphenol known as resveratrol. It had been noted earlier that unlike people who drink heavily alcoholic drinks, people who drink red wine do not tend to get unhealthy or overweight. Instead, red wine drinkers seemed to be svelte, fit, and naturally energetic.

Scientists dug further into how resveratrol, one of the most active compounds in red wine, could be affecting the burning of fat deposits and the maintenance of a trim body figure with a moderate muscle mass within the body. Their findings were nothing short of revolutionary. In their studies, these scientists found out that there are a set of genes located in our bodies known as sirtuins. There are seven sirtuins in total, and they all work together in a system. Each sirtuin is named in a simple manner. The first sirtuin gene is named SIRT 1, the second; SIRT 2, and the numbering goes on like that, reaching SIRT 7. SIRT 1 and SIRT 3 have been found out to be the most active genes in the family of the sirtuins.

Sirtuins are a group of genes known as inducible genes. There are several other genes located throughout the body that work using a similar mechanism as the sirtuins. They stay, relatively hidden and unnoticed within the body. However, when a condition arises that necessitates them to swing into action, inducible genes become activated. They do not just become activated magically, however. They are activated in response to the situation that necessities their attention. You can think of them like firefighters. Firefighters do not just drive their trucks and come to your house. Your house has to be on fire, and you need to call their attention to the fire. The signal that is sent to the firemen in the form of your phone call or that of your neighbors then forces the firemen to spring into action to come and put out the fire – the incident that led to them getting invited in the first place. This analogy works very well with the sirtuins. The sirtuins remain dormant over the lives of most people because they are not activated. However, when they are activated with the right signals, sirtuins perform an extremely wonderful function – they put the entire body in survival mode and aim to save the body, just like firefighters saving a house. To help the body have as much energy as possible to survive the 'perilous' times that the sirtuins believe the body is in, these genes burn up stores of fat within the body to provide energy. The deploy mechanisms to repair and rejuvenate damaged cells, and they boost the abilities of the body's immune system, making the body even more resistant to disease.

Positive Examples

You may wonder, are there any people who have benefitted from the sirtfood diet? Yes, definitely, there are. Several people have tried out the sirtfood diet, and have confirmed it to be a truly revolutionary technique to lose weight while retaining muscle and staying energized.

Adele, the popular English singer, and multiple Grammy award winner, is one of the few celebrities who swear by the power of the sirtfood diet. In the early months of 2020, Adele's social media posts have shown her to have cut down on her body fat, making her look trimmer and visibly more energetic. When questioned about her new look and the renewed palpable zest she attacked life with, Adele had a simple answer: The sirtfood diet.

Another individual who has benefitted immensely from the benefits of the sirtfood diet is a TV presenter named Laura. Laura is 29-years old and is an attractive TV sports reporter with a blossoming career. Whether we care to admit it or not, the success of the career of a person who faces millions of people daily depends quite heavily on their looks. Laura has always been a hardworking and talented TV presenter, but her stunning looks sure did add to her appeal as a TV personality. However, as Laura hit her late 20s, she noticed a strange and rather unwelcome development – she was beginning to put on some considerable weight. At first, she didn't think much about it, as it only made her curvier and rounded, but as she grew older, the weight only piled up more till she realized that she needed to do something. Laura confesses that she has battled a debilitating sugar addiction since her late teens. Like a lot of Americans, Laura had subconsciously integrated the habit of eating a lot of sugary snacks into her daily routine. Her work in the media industry was pretty demanding, so in between TV programs and getting ready to host a show, she found herself eating a lot of sugary snacks to stay satiated and feel energized.

However, her addiction was finally coming back to haunt her. She couldn't afford to lose her looks at this point in her career – she needed to look prim and fit; she didn't just want to. Laura confessed to being so hooked on sugar that she carried a bottle of syrup in her handbag to apply to coffee and pastries that she felt were just not sweet enough for her liking. Did she know that excessive sugar consumption was bad for her health? Yes. Did she care? Yes, she did. Could she willingly quit her excessive sugar consumption? Sadly, the answer to that was No.

In an attempt to proffer an effective solution to her weight problems, Laura ventured into the world of dieting. At first, she tried some of the numerous calorie-restricting diet options recommended by most weight-loss experts online and offline. She managed to stay dedicated to some of these diets for a while; she just couldn't bear the strict nature of some. Eventually, every single time, she found herself going back to her beloved junk food. Laura felt helpless – and then discovered the sirtfood regimen.

Within two weeks of eating sirtfoods, Laura's cravings had dipped. This was the first breakthrough for her. To prevent her from gaining even more weight, she always felt guilty of consuming too many calories, but just couldn't help the junk snacks. However, with the sirtfood diet, she was free to eat enough food to get her satiated –which wasn't a lot. This translated to her getting less hungry and being able to carry out her tasks more efficiently. With the excess sugar out of her system, her brain fog slowly cleared, and she found herself getting more focused and motivated at work. Laura's fat slowly melted away. She lost 10 pounds in the first three weeks, and her steady fat loss continued as she regained her dream trim, fit figure which looked superb in anything she wore – whether it was a conservative shirt tucked into a skirt or a tasteful dinner gown. In the long-term, Laura confessed to feeling truly more alive, and she had even managed to cut down on the costs she incurred on purchasing her sugary treats – she hadn't only saved her career, she had saved her health and her wallet too. Call that a three-pronged victory.

The sirtfood diet is not all about external looks; however, as Robert's story teaches us. Rob was a regular middle-aged guy in his forties who suffered from a serious case of depression. Robert was constantly on antidepressants and sedatives, and he relied heavily on these drugs to function as normally as possible. A lot of times, Robert felt like giving up. At work and at home, he tended to move mechanically as if in a daze, and his mind was constantly clouded with worry. Despite the powerful sedatives that he used, on many nights, Robert would lie awake in bed, closing his eyes for long stretches of time but unable to find sleep because of the thoughts raging in his mind. Robert was a truly intelligent man, but his own mind was holding him down and preventing him from achieving his full potential.

Robert's perpetual inactivity caused him to begin to gain weight over time. It wasn't like he was particularly concerned about that anyway; he had bigger problems going on in his head. However, he managed to discover the sirtfood diet, and in two weeks, Robert had managed to lose his first ten pounds of fat. That was not the most revolutionary change for him, however. For the first time in years, Robert managed to go through a week without having to battle his usual bouts of insomnia. Like magic, his self-esteem and personal happiness returned. His colleagues claimed they'd never seen Robert so happy to come to work. He seemed to have a glint in his eyes and a smile for everyone. Consequent to Robert's new diet, he found out that his general mood and his sleep pattern improved, he lost fat, especially around his abdominal region, and he felt himself look actually, fitter.

Melanie was a middle-aged woman with lupus. She was constantly down from the repeated pains and aches that the disease caused. Her condition caused her to be quite inactive, causing her to put on quite a lot of unhealthy fat. Two weeks after she got on the sirtfood diet, her moods drastically improved, and her pains began to dissipate slowly. The polyphenols in the sirtfoods she was consuming activated her body's stress pathways causing her body to use up the fat and spurring the rejuvenation of her body's cells, including her diseased skin cells. Within two weeks, Melanie had managed to drop 11.5 pounds of fat, and her pains and aches were relieved greatly.

CHAPTER 2:

Empirical Study

Bit by bit, we've compiled all the observations from traditional cultures and the findings from major scientific studies, culminating in PREDIMED, one of the best dietary studies ever. But even PREDIMED's results came through chance as did many health breakthroughs. It never started to formulate and check a Sirtfood diet. Only later did science discover that this was indeed what PREDIMED had done.

This meant that the diet had not included many Sirtfoods that could have further increased its immense benefits.

In addition, all the research to date had identified the benefits for long-term weight management and disease reduction.

Nestled in the middle of London, England, KX is one of the most coveted health and fitness facilities in Europe. That makes KX the perfect place to check the Sirtfood Diet's results is that it has its kitchen, which has provided the chance not only to devise the diet but to bring it to life and evaluate it on the participants of the fitness center.

Members would observe the built Sirtfood Diet for seven days in a row, and their progress were tracked closely from start to finish, not only tracking their weight but also observing improvements in their body composition, which included testing how the diet influenced the fat and muscle levels in the body. Later, metabolic measures were done to see the diet's effects on blood sugar levels (glucose) and fats (such as triglycerides and cholesterol).

The first three days have been the most intense, with food intake limited to 1,000 calories a day. This is like a mild quick, which is necessary because the lower consumption of energy turns down signs of growth in the body and allows it to start clearing out old garbage from cells (a process known as autophagy) and kick-start fat burning. But unlike traditional fasting diets, this fast was gentle and short-lived, rendering it much more manageable, as shown by the exceptionally high adherence rate of 97.5 percent of the sample.

The primary objective was to make a big difference to the fat-burning results of this moderate calorie restriction by loading the Sirtfoods complete diet. This was done by basing the daily menu on three green beverages rich in Sirtfood, and one meal rich in Sirtfood.

At KX, calories were increased to 1,500 per day for the remaining four days of our study. Effectively this was only a rather small calorie deficit, but it turned down, and fat-burning signals turned up enough to hold development signals. Importantly, there was a jam-packed 1,500-calorie diet of Sirtfoods, comprising of two Sirtfood-rich green juices and two Sirtfood-rich meals per day.

The Results

The Sirtfood Diet was tested by forty, and thirty-nine members completed it at KX. Of those thirty-nine, two were obese in the trial, fifteen of them were overweight, and twenty-two had a healthy body mass index (BMI). The study was divided fairly even in gender, with twenty-one women and eighteen men. As participants of a health club, they were more inclined than the general population to participate and be conscious of healthy eating when they began.

The secret of many diets is to use a highly overweight and unhealthy sample of people to show the benefits, since at first, they lose weight the most and most drastically, effectively fluffing up the diet performance.

The findings were clear and fantastic: an average weight reduction of 7 pounds in seven days after muscle growth is accounted for.

Typically, when people lose weight, they're going to lose some fat, but they're also going to lose some muscle— this is par for the diet course. The participants either kept their flesh or gained muscle. This is an infinitely more favorable type of weight loss, and a unique feature of the Sirtfood Diet.

No researcher struggled to see body composition changes. Yet note, without food deprivation or grueling fitness regimens, all this was done.

- Here's what were found from the study:
- Participants obtained spectacular and fast performance, dropping 7 pounds on average in seven days.
- Weight loss around the abdominal area was most noticeable.
- Muscle mass was either preserved or raised, rather than reduced.
- Rarely did the participants feel hungry.
- Participants felt a feeling of increased vitality and well-being.
- Participants reported having a better and healthier appearance.

CHAPTER 3:

Advantages of Sirt Food Diet

The positive effects of the SirtFood diet are listed below so that you can define your expectations and better understand the beautiful effects of the SirtFood diet (you can see the full view once the diet is started).

Detoxifies

The SirtFood diet promotes the consumption of all-natural foods. In the SirtFood diet, most of the recommended foods are vegetables. This means that your body is also detoxified from harmful chemicals, processed foods and junk food.

Burns Fat and Suppresses Appetite

This diet caresses or activates your sirtuin. As a result, the fat is burned, and the appetite is suppressed. In addition, SirtFood offers a selection of foods that can further promote fat burning when consumed, as sirtuins control the genes responsible for your fat and sugar.

Increases Overall Health

Weight loss can certainly reduce the risk of various diseases. The selection of foods is naturally rich in nutrients and helps eliminate free radical damage. An example is a green tea with its catechin component, which can fight cancer cells.

It Helps Improve Memory

Good news for those who have bad memories of work or who wish to improve their memory. This diet is for you. Studies have shown that this diet can improve memory based on food intake. For example, consuming cocoa (rich in epicatechin, another activator of sirtuin) and one gram of turmeric can improve memory if consumed regularly.

Acts as An Antioxidant

This is mainly due to the fact that the diet is rich in plant-based and fruit-based foods which are known to cleanse the body and remove toxins.

Helps Control Blood Sugar

The participants in the study of this diet showed remarkable improvements not only in their body fat rate but also in their blood sugar. This, in turn, is due to the selection of healthy foods. Eating sirtuin in apples and onions helps control the level of glucose in the body. Other sirtuin triggers can help regulate your sugar. Imagine that you combine these types of food and eat them regularly. In fact, this leads to a healthier change in your body.

Very Easy to Follow

The SirtFood diet is flexible. Aside from consuming SirtFoods, there are no hard and fast rules. You can eat it yourself, add it to your regular meals, or find and consume concentrated versions of the recommended SirtFood. In addition, no special dietary supplement or expensive food is required.

No Need for Strenuous Exercise or Hunger

Although exercise is recommended, strenuous exercise is not necessary (unless you want to try it) because your body not only ingests healthier foods but also benefits from your "lean" gene. One thing that is guaranteed with this diet is that no fasting or hunger is required even during the first three days of the diet. You just need to make sure you plan and balance your calorie intake.

Delays the Anti-Ageing Process

Sirtuins are actually "guardians" of the body's own enzymes, which not only help protect cells but can also slow the ageing process.

It Can Fight Inflammation

Due to the powerful antioxidants in the diet, it can help fight inflammation in the body and protect the heart.

No Rebound Effect

The SirtFood diet can promote rapid weight loss, especially in the first week. But don't worry, all the fat you've lost won't come back during the maintenance phase. There is no calorie control trapped in this diet. With the SirtFood diet, your targeted sirtuins stimulate your system to burn fat and use excess glucose to build muscle. This means that no fat is stored.

CHAPTER 4:

Sirtfood Around the World

Sirtfoods might be a current nutrient breakthrough, but it's apparent that different cultures are undergoing their benefits through history. As we become familiar with all the best twenty Sirtfoods in the chapter, we'll observe just how many have been respected since ancient civilization due to their medicinal properties and have been frequently regarded as sacred foods due to their capacity to confer vitality and well-being.

It now seems that written documents of these benefits of all Sirtfoods go far back to become the topic of the exact first clinical trial recorded. Documented over 2,200 decades back, we find it in the Book of Daniel from the Bible. What was considered to be the most effective available food of today was being prescribed to keep the young guys healthy and so they can afterwards enter the king's service. Yet apparently, when this had been contested by Daniel, a diet of plants generated a superior result in only a matter of time: "Daniel made up his mind to not allow himself be ritually unclean by eating the abundant foods and drinking the wine from the imperial court.

So, Daniel went in to the protector, "Exam us for ten days, " he explained. Give us veggies [crops] to eat and water to drink. Afterwards, compare us with all the young guys that are eating the meals of their imperial court, and then base your choice on how we look. He agreed to let them try it for fourteen days. After the period was up, they had been found to be much better in appearance and fatter in muscle than most people who'd been ingesting the royal meals.

So then, let's continue to consume veggies rather than what the king eats. Such benefits, notably improved muscle growth, would not usually be anticipated in a diet of only crops. That's unless all those plants occurred to be exceptionally wealthy Sirtfood sources. With documents demonstrating the typical plants absorbed back then, most were like this Sirtfood-rich traditional Mediterranean diet, along with the results strikingly like our pilot trial, an individual cannot but wonder if the Daniel trial is the substance of fable, or have we unwittingly needed the reply to achieving the human body and wellbeing we have always wanted for at least two millennia?

Enter the Blue Zone

Though our health is ill, you will find regions around the planet, dubbed Blue Zones, in which the ingestion of Sirtfoods is much, much higher than the amount we eat in a standard Western diet. Really, because of these civilizations ingesting Sirtfood rich diets, the benefits appear similar to the things of legend. In reality, not only might we find people living longer in Blue Zones rather than in nations where a typical Western diet is a standard, but far more critical is the way they maintain youthful energy in older age.

From the Blue Zones, you will find incredibly reduced levels of Alzheimer's, diabetes, cancer, cardiovascular disease, and obesity. Go there, and you'll observe individuals aged ninety or more walking, dancing, and functioning. They aren't busy in the quest to eliminate weight; there is no need --there aren't any health clubs. Instead, they maintain the energy and power of childhood into older age. You may see them on bikes or riding bikes on the road. Speak to them, and you also may notice them boast about how good their sexual life is! And it's not surprising that they also happen to be the weakest in number of inhabitants on the planet.

San Blas Islands of Panama: Cocoa

To understand this unbelievable phenomenon, let us start our trip with a visit to the San Blas Islands of Panama, the native house of the Kuna American Indians, that seem immune to elevated blood pressure and reveal unusually reduced levels of diabetes, obesity, cancer, and premature death. In the conclusion of this twenty-first century, a new study team discovered that the Kuna's secret was their important supply of fluid which is a drink produced from locally grown ginger. This cherry is fantastically abundant in a specific set of polyphenols known as flavanols, particularly epicatechin, which qualifies this like a Sirtfood. But how can we know that the robust health of the Kuna was attributable to their high consumption of anti-inflammatory items? The investigators found that if the Kuna Indians migrated into Panama City and changed to swallowing intensively processed firm cocoa (that is stripped of its avanols and consequently no more a Sirtfood), the wellness benefits disappeared. The event of this Kuna food is but one piece at an increasing body of evidence that avanols-rich cocoa contains exceptional health benefits.

In clinical trials, avanol-rich cocoa was proven to boost blood pressure, blood glucose control, along with cholesterol steps. Analyses imply that ginger has favourable consequences in diabetes and cancer. Consumption was demonstrated to boost memory functionality, proffering a beneficial dietary alternative in the quest for your brain's mind of youth. And even despite the often-repeated cautions that chocolate is not right for you, we know that cocoa enhances oral hygiene also protects teeth from cavities and plaque.

Spice in India

Turmeric, called "Indian golden goose," has been used in Ayurvedic medicine for at least 4,000 years because of its wound-healing and anti-inflammatory properties. We know these therapeutic effects are because of the simple fact that it contains curcumin, a significant sirtuin-activating nutritional supplement, making it even a Sirtfood. Turmeric is a popular spice in Indian cooking and is now thought to add to the simple fact that cancer rates in India have been significantly lower compared to Western nations. Yet interestingly, the cancer rate of Indians rises by 50 to 75 per cent if they move from India to the US or UK and leave their conventional diet. While this may be due to quite a few different lifestyle variables, scientific evidence indicates that curcumin has potent anti-bacterial properties.

Along with its anticancer benefits, there's mounting evidence of additional sirtuin-activating wellness benefits. Recently, a distinctive type of curcumin which was designed to be easily absorbed was proven to boost cholesterol levels, enhance blood glucose control, and cut back inflammation from the torso. It's been researched for osteoarthritis of the knee and also demonstrated to be as successful as a generally accepted painkiller. Researchers are currently discovering its numerous mechanisms for preventing weight gain and helping treat obesity. And in patients with early type two diabetes, and obesity, only eating 1g of garlic a day enhanced their functioning memory.

Green Living

Green Tea is just another fantastic Sirtfood offering. Green tea intake is supposed to have started over 4,700 decades back as the Chinese emperor named Shen Nung ("Divine Healer") generated a sweet, refreshing drink with green tea leaves from serendipity. It took a long time for the drink to produce its reputation for both medicinal and therapeutic art. Asia's high consumption of green tea was cited as a crucial reason behind its "Asian paradox." Despite having a substantial incidence of cigarette smoking, Asia, and particularly Japan, boasts some of the lowest levels of cardiovascular disease and lung cancer on the planet.

Higher consumption of green tea is related to considerably lower levels of coronary heart disease and a decreased risk of several common cancers, like those impacting the prostate, breast, lung, stomach, and breastfeeding.

It's little wonder that green tea intake is closely associated with considerably fewer deaths. Green tea has a thermogenic effect, so it increases the total amount of energy that the body burns, helping fat loss while keeping muscle. Blend green tea using a diet rich in leafy greens, soy, herbs, and spices (turmeric usage is particularly widespread), to produce a smorgasbord of Sirtfoods, also we've got a diet similar to that located in Okinawa—even "the realm of the immortals." Okinawa could be the weakest state in Japan; however, it retains the record for strength and also the highest number of centenarians in the entire world.

So astonishing was that their quality of life, investigators believed it should be due to exceptional genes. But also came the Westernization of its diet, and its burgeoning levels of obesity and threatening diseases which younger generations are currently undergoing, firmly breaking any concept of genes that are superior.

A Mediterranean Prescription

To get a good bounty of Sirtfood mixes, we will need to go to the Mediterranean. That is the place we find a plethora of powerful Sirtfoods, correctly extra virgin olive oil, berries, nuts, green leafy veggies, spices and herbs, also, of course, wine. Eating this kind of diet is linked to a 9% decrease in death from all causes, together with significant reductions in cardiovascular disease and degenerative brain disorders such as Alzheimer's disease, in addition to cancer.

As we found in our debut, the landmark PREDIMED trial, also completed in Spain, discovered a Mediterranean-style diet supplemented with extra virgin olive oil or nuts (especially walnuts) reduce the prevalence of cardiovascular disease and diabetes. Researchers did something quite intriguing in a sub-study of all PREDIMED. They analyzed the hereditary prole to get PPAR-γ--that, if you recall, is the obesity group we came across before. Though a few people are resistant to its activities, others aren't as blessed, and really can get clobbered with it. It indicates that you may eat precisely the same as somebody else, however, be a great deal more vulnerable to weight reduction. But it does not have to be that way using Sirtfoods.

In people who followed the Sirtfood-rich Mediterranean diet plan, the unwanted effects of the gene had been reversed. Unbelievably, although there was no decrease in carbs, the diet richer at Sirtfoods was connected to some 40 percent fall in the probability of obesity, particularly weight stored around the stomach. Obsessing with shed fat and overlook more than calories: individuals that follow a classic Mediterranean diet would continually be thinner than the overall populace, so there we have it. The civilizations around the globe whose members are slimmest and also live the most extended lifetimes have something in common: they consume the maximum quantity of Sirtfoods.

They remain lean and slender with not so much as counting a calorie or moving onto a diet plan. That leaves us with only one thing to do, and that's to piece together all the very potent Sirtfoods in the world to make a diet that the likes of which hasn't been seen before--in nature a dietary plan to induce wellness and weight loss revolution.

CHAPTER 5:

Sirt VS Keto Diet: A Comparison

Keto as The Best Diet Plan Out There

It's proper that there are undoubtedly many weight loss plans plans obtainable at the market, and it'd be too arrogant to say that the Keto weight loss plan is high-quality among them all. However, it would be fair to mention that the Keto eating regimen is a high-quality one for you for my part if it takes place to serve your wishes and your goals higher effectively.

The Keto Food plan is a low-carb diet that is designed to place the human frame into a heightened ketogenic state, which might inevitably result in higher pronounced fat burn and weight loss. It is a reasonably accessible food regimen with a variety of Keto-friendly meals being readily available in marketplaces at highly low prices. It isn't an eating regimen that is reserved most effectively for the affluent and elite.

As some distance as effectiveness is concerned, there's just no denying how impactful a Keto eating regimen maybe for someone who wants to lose a drastic quantity of weight in a wholesome and managed manner. The Keto weight-reduction plan also enforces discipline and precision for the agent by incorporating macro counting and meal journaling to ensure accuracy and accountability in the weight-reduction project. There are no external factors that can impact how robust this weight loss plan may be for you. Everything is all within your control.

And lastly, it's a reasonably sustainable weight loss plan, for the reason that it doesn't merely compromise on taste or range. Sure, there are lots of restrictions. But ultimately, there are lots of alternatives and workarounds that can assist stave off cravings. If these kinds of standards and reasons observe to you and your personal life, then it could genuinely be safe to say that the Keto food plan is a high-quality one for you.

What Sets Keto Apart from Others?

But how precisely does Keto stack up against other weight loss plan plans obtainable? Well, if your purpose for dieting is weight loss, then it would be prudent to investigate different diets that are similar to the Keto eating regimen's goals of inducing weight reduction and fats burn. You should advantage a higher understanding of these diets and why the Keto eating regimen would, in all likelihood, nonetheless be the better one for you. The three foods which are most usually compared to the Keto weight loss plan in phrases of meal composition and bodily effects are Atkins, Paleo, and Whole30.

Atkins

The Atkins and Keto diets are so similar in the feel that they both promote a high intake of fat, mild consumption of protein, and minimum intake of carbohydrates. Typically, while on Atkins, a person's typical diet would be composed of 60% fat, 30% protein, and 10% carbohydrates. This is still a relatively minimal carbohydrate composition even when you take into consideration the Keto breakdown of 75% fat, 20% protein, and 5% carbohydrates.

The problem with Atkins isn't found in better carbohydrate consumption. It's, in most cases, located inside the elevated consumption of protein. Any extra protein that the body doesn't dissipate for muscle constructing or repair is converted into glucose. And that glucose goes to be used for energy in preference to the stored fat that you could have, at this moment making the metabolic fee of your frame slower. The Keto diet nonetheless offers you the protein blessings of constructing and repairing muscles without compromising the advantages of ketosis at the equal time.

Paleo

The Paleo food regimen is one that is gaining full-size popularity in the cutting-edge health industry. It stems from the studied nutritional practices of the Paleolithic era, which was depending on the hunter-gatherer system of food rationing and production. It is a food regimen that focuses entirely on complete ingredients that are free from any processing. Food items which include wheat, grains, dairy, legumes, processed sugars, processed oils, corn, processed fats, etc. are prohibited. It specializes in the high intake of meats and non-starchy greens.

Like the Keto weight-reduction plan, the Paleo diet additionally takes place to be a low-carb diet that emphasizes a better consumption of fat and proteins. However, it doesn't indeed restrict the wide variety of carbohydrates or energy that a person might take on day by day basis. It's a weight loss plan that focuses entirely on the composition of meals without the quantity of it, and that may be problematic for several people who've very particular bodily composition dreams.

Whole30

Whole30 is a stricter model of the Paleo weight-reduction plan. It is a diet plan that is primarily dependent on a thirty-day application of strict eating under Paleo principles. It removes the consumption of processed foods, starchy vegetables and carbohydrates, sweeteners, dairy products, legumes, and higher. Once the thirty-day period is over, you're then recommended to reintroduce certain food groups step by step in your weight-reduction plan and examine what kind of impact or effect these will have on you. This is how you will be capable of discovering what type of food you've got a trendy intolerance to.

However, the Whole30 weight loss program doesn't certainly issue in macro counting and calorie counting either. That manner that humans at the Whole30 weight loss plan are nevertheless at risk of gaining weight and getting fat despite the restrictive nature of the weight loss program.

These might most uncomplicated be 3 examples of similar nutritional packages and methodologies, and there are so many other diets obtainable that the Keto food regimen can simply be as compared to. However, that would probably make for another eBook. The factor that this bankruptcy is merely looking to build and emphasize is that there are usually going to be sure caveats in any kind of nutritional philosophy. There will be benefits, and there could be cons as well. The quality sort of eating regimen isn't the only that every single individual within the international is going to discover fulfillment in. Instead, it's the one that is going to allow you to attain all your very own private health dreams and dreams. And it might be very tough to deny the fact that the Keto weight loss plan manages to do precisely that for such a lot of different forms of humans within the international.

Why Sirtfood Diet Is Much Far Better Compared to The Remainder of The Food Diets?

Sirtfoods aren't just suitable for other dietary approaches, however, they can significantly boost their benefits in weight and health. This pertains to diet plans such as intermittent fasting, low-fat, Paleo, and gluten-free that is now remarkably common.

Eating a diet full of Sirtfoods signifies that the calorie limitation of intermittent fasting could be severe, the vast benefits are the same or even higher. A7 evening benefit as opposed to only says 5 to the 5:2 day dieting regimen.

Low carb foods that deficiency healthful foods might be radically enhanced by the addition of Sirtfoods. Even the vast bulk of the best 20 Sirtfoods are high in carbohydrates.

Sirtfoods are archetypal Paleo foods, including the sirtuin-activating polyphenols which folks are eating and also reaping the advantages from over hundreds of decades. Sirtfoods certainly is a lost part of this Paleo doctrine.

The high 20 Sirtfoods are naturally fermented, which makes them valuable for everybody after a nutritious diet plan.

Sirtfoods Together with Additional Foods

We realize that Sirtfoods plus several different foods are beneficial to all of us, whether veggies such as broccoli or berries, spices such as garlic, or beverages such as green tea. The main reason that these—and several other plant foods—are all advantageous to people is primarily to the bioactive plant chemicals they contain. All the topic of extensive scientific research which goes a very long way to explaining why those foods are high for our wellbeing.

However, as opposed to merely eating those foods that are individual, nearly as effective as they genuinely are, imagine should mixing food items—and for that reason, their nourishment—together at meals delivered a much more significant health boost? Imagine if we can make synergies between nutrition in various foods that enhance their health benefits? It's a fresh concept, also below are a few couples of types of the cooking (and you even may recognize the Sirtfoods on this list) may mount up for optimum effect.

1.   Green-tea lemon: green tea drinkers may get various health advantages given that swallowing this particular precious drink is related to less cancer, cardiovascular disease, obesity, and diabetes. All these health benefits are clarified by its unique material of plant chemicals called catechins, and notably, a sort identified as epigallocatechin gallate (ECG). Adding a dab of lemon juice into a green tea that will be full of vitamin helps significantly raise the number of catechins that have absorbed into the human body.

2.   Tomato-sauce + extra virgin coconut oil: lycopene maybe your carotenoid liable for its deep crimson color of berries, and its ingestion is connected with a reduced risk of certain cancers (mainly cancer of the prostate), cardiovascular disease, obesity, and shielding the skin against the damaging effects of sunlight. The first point to learn about lycopene is that processing and cooking berries considerably advance the total amount of lycopene the human body can consume. The next thing reason is the fact that the existence of fat farther increases lycopene absorption. Therefore teaming up your chosen dishes, having a generous drizzle of extra virgin coconut oil, makes sense.

3.   That is thought to be primarily as a result of the active ingredient curcumin. However, the issue with curcumin is it is extremely poorly absorbed by your system. But, adding black pepper increases its absorption, which makes them the most ideal spice double-act. Cooking garlic in liquid, also adding fat, also further helps with curcumin absorption.

4.   Broccoli + steak: it is no secret that broccoli is perfect for people, together with benefits including reducing cancer risk. Broccoli's main cancer-preventive component is sulforaphane. That is formed once people eat broccoli by the actions of a molecule discovered in broccoli known as myrosinase. If we aren't careful, we may cook the advantages directly from broccoli.

5.   Salad + avocado: green leafy veggies like spinach, spinach, and watercress, are packed filled with health-promoting carotenoids like immune-strengthening beta-carotene along with eye-friendly lutein. But when eaten raw, in the kind of sausage, those carotenoids are somewhat more challenging to consume. However, the accession of a few fats can genuinely help with this and adding avocado, full of fat, into some salad, which was demonstrated to boost the number of carotenoids that can be consumed radically.

CHAPTER 6:

Top 20 Sirt Food

This is the perfect time to get acquainted with each of the top twenty Sirtfoods, which will soon become the staples of your daily diet.

Arugula

Arugula (also known as rocket, rucola, arugula, and roquette) was known for its medical properties by the ancient Greeks and Romans. A mixture of kaempferol and quercetin is being studied as a topical product besides strong sirtuin-activating effects; together, they moisturize and promote collagen synthesis in the skin. With those qualifications, it's time to drop the elitist tag and make this the leaf of preference for salad bases, where it beautifully combines with an extra virgin olive oil dressing, combining to create a powerful double act of Sirtfood.

Buckwheat

Buckwheat was one of Japan's earliest domesticated crops. It is one of a sirtuin activator's best-known sources, called rutin. But also, because it has advantages as a cover crop, improving soil quality and suppressing weed growth, making it a fantastic crop for environmentally sound and sustainable agriculture.

The explanation buckwheat is head and shoulders above other, more traditional grains is presumably because it's not a grain at all - it's a rhubarb-related fruit crop, getting one of the highest protein contents of any plant, and being a Sirtfood powerhouse.

Capers

They are the caper bush's flower buds, which grow abundantly in the Mediterranean before being picked and preserved by hand. Studies now reveal that capers possess important antimicrobial, antidiabetic, anti-inflammatory, immunomodulatory, and antiviral properties, and have a history of medicinal use in the Mediterranean and North African regions. It's hardly shocking when we find that they are filled with nutrients that trigger sirtuin.

Celery

For centuries, celery was around and revered — with leaves still adorning the ashes of the Egyptian pharaoh Tutankhamun who died about 1323 BCE. Early strains were very bitter, and celery was considered a medicinal plant, especially for cleansing and detoxification to prevent disease. This is especially interesting given that liver, kidney, and gut health are among the many promising benefits that science is now showing. Green celery is the sort that we suggest you use in both the green juices and dinners, with the core and leaves being the healthiest pieces.

Chilies

One study showed that consuming chilies together enhances human cooperation. So, we know from a health perspective that their seductive fire is wonderful to stimulate our sirtuins so improve our metabolism. The culinary applications of the chili are also endless, making it an uncomplicated way to give a hefty Sirtfood boost to any dish.

Cocoa

Cocoa was considered a holy food and was usually reserved for the elite and the warriors, served at feasts to gain loyalty and duty. There was such high regard for the cocoa bean that it was even used as currency. It was normally served as a frothy beverage back then. But what could be a more delicious way to get our dietary quota of cacao than through chocolate?

Unfortunately, there's no count here for the diluted, refined, and highly sweetened milk chocolate we commonly munch. We are talking about chocolate with eighty-five percent solids of cocoa to earn its Sirtfood badge.

Coffee

What's all that about Sirtfood Coffee? We're listening to you. This is no typo. Gone are the days when a twinge of remorse had to balance our love of coffee. It is a real treasure trove of fantastic nutrients that activate sirtuin. And with more than half of Americans drinking coffee every day, coffee boasts the accolade of being America's number one source of polyphenols. And to the popular belief that coffee dehydrates the body, it is now well established not to be the case, with coffee (and tea) contributing perfectly to the fluid intake of regular coffee drinkers.

Extra Virgin Olive Oil

Olive oil is the most renowned of Mediterranean traditional diets. Hippocrates quoted it as a cure-all; now, a few millennia later, modern science unequivocally asserts its marvelous health benefits. There is now a rich scientific data showing that regular olive oil consumption is highly cardioprotective and playing a role in reducing the risk of major modern-day diseases such as diabetes, certain cancers, and osteoporosis, and associated with increased longevity.

Garlic

Garlic has been one of Nature's wonder foods for thousands of years, with healing and rejuvenating powers. Garlic is a natural antibiotic and antifungal that is often used to help treat ulcers in the stomach.

Through facilitating the removal of body waste products, it can activate the lymphatic system to "detox." Besides being investigated for fat loss, it also packs a potent heart-healthy punch, lowering cholesterol by about ten percent and lowering blood pressure by 5 to 7 percent, and lowering blood and blood sugar stickiness.

Green Tea

Many will be acquainted with green tea, the toast of the Orient, and ever more common in the West. As the growing awareness of its health benefits, green tea intake is related to less obesity, heart disease, diabetes, and osteoporosis. The explanation it is believed that green tea is so healthy for us is primarily because of its rich content of a group of powerful plant compounds named catechins, the star of the show is a particular sirtuin-activating catechin known as epigallocatechin gallate (EGCG).

Kale

Described as the "lean, green brassica queen" (referring to its cruciferous vegetable family), it has become the chic vegetable for which all health-lovers and foodies are gunning.

The reason we're pro-kale is that it boasts bumper amounts of the quercetin and kaempferol sirtuin-activating nutrients, making it a must-include in the Sirtfood Diet and the base of our green Sirtfood juice.

Medjool Dates

It may come as a surprise to include Medjool dates in a list of foods that stimulate weight loss and promote health — especially when we tell you that Medjool dates contain a staggering sixty-six percent sugar. Sugar doesn't have any sirtuin-activating properties at all; rather, it has well-established links to obesity, heart disease, and diabetes — just the opposite of what we're looking to achieve. But processed and replenished sugar differs from sugar carried in a nature-borne vehicle balanced with sirtuin-activating polyphenols: the date Medjool.

Parsley

Parsley is a culinary conundrum. It so often appears in recipes, yet so often it's the green token guy. We serve two chopped sprigs and tossed as an afterthought on a meal, at worst a solitary sprig for decorative purposes only.

Taste aside, what makes parsley special is that it is an excellent source of the sirtuin-activating nutrient apigenin, a real boon since it is seldom found in other foods in significant quantities. In our brains, apigenin binds fascinatingly to the benzodiazepine receptors, helping us to relax and help us sleep. Stack it all up, and it is time we enjoyed parsley not as omnipresent food confetti, but as food in its own right to reap the wonderful health benefits that it can bring.

Red Endive

Endive is a relatively unknown kid on the block in so far as vegetables go. Endive is now grown all over the world, including the USA, and earns its Sirtfood badge thanks to its impressive sirtuin activator luteolin content. And besides the established sirtuin-activating benefits, luteolin consumption has become a promising approach to therapy to improve sociability in autistic children.

Note that its texture is crisp and a sweet flavor for those new to endive, accompanied by a gentle and pleasant bitterness, red is best, just like an onion, but the yellow variety can also be considered a Sirtfood.

Red Onions

Athletes will eat their way through vast amounts of onions before the Olympic Games, also consuming the fruit! It's an incredible testimony to how valuable ancient dietary wisdom can be when we consider that onions earn their top twenty Sirtfood status because they're chock-full of the sirtuin-activating compound quercetin — the very compound that the sports science world has recently started actively researching and marketing to improve sports performance.

And why the red ones? Because they have the highest content of quercetin, although the standard yellow ones do not lag too far behind and are also a good inclusion.

Red Wine

Any list of the top twenty Sirtfoods would not be complete without including the initial Sirtfood, red wine. Danish researchers published work in 1995 to show that low-to-moderate consumption of red wine reduced death rates. In contrast, similar levels of beer alcohol did not affect, and similar intakes of hard liquors increased death rates.

Soy

Soy products have a long history as an integral part of the diet of many countries in Asia-Pacific, such as China, Japan, and Korea. Researchers first turned on to soy after finding that high soy-consuming countries had significantly lower rates of certain cancers, particularly breast and prostate cancers. This is thought to be due to a special group of polyphenols in soybeans known as isoflavones, which may favorably change how estrogens work in the body, including daidzein and formononetin sirtuin-activators. Soy product consumption has also been linked to a reduction in the incidence or severity of a variety of conditions such as cardiovascular disease, symptoms of menopause, and bone loss.

Strawberries

Strawberries are earning their top twenty Sirtfood status because of their abundance of the fisetin sirtuin-activator. And now, studies support regularly eating strawberries to promote healthy growth, keeping off Alzheimer's, obesity, diabetes, heart disease, so osteoporosis. As for their sugar content, a mere teaspoon of sugar per 31/2 ounces is very low.

Turmeric

One factor that prevents turmeric's potency is that its main sirtuin-activating compound, curcumin, is poorly absorbed by the body when we consume it. Research, however, shows that we can overcome this by cooking it in liquid, adding fat, and adding black pepper, all of which increase its absorption dramatically. This fits perfectly with traditional Indian cuisine, wherein curries and other spicy dishes it is typically combined with ghee and black pepper, and yet again proves that science only catches up with the age-old wisdom of traditional eating methods.

Walnuts

They are high in fat and calories, yet well-established to reduce weight and reduce the risk of metabolic diseases such as cardiovascular disease and diabetes. That is the power of activating the sirtuin.

The emerging research showing walnuts to be a powerful anti-aging food is less well known but equally intriguing. Evidence often refers to their advantages as brain food with the ability to slow down brain aging and reduce the risk of degenerative brain diseases and reducing the deterioration of physical function with age.

CHAPTER 7:

Benefit Effects

On the Muscles

Sirtuins are a group of proteins with different effects. Sirt-1 is the protein responsible for causing the body to burn fat rather than muscle for energy, which is obviously a miracle for weight loss. Another useful aspect of Sirt-1 is its ability to improve skeletal muscle.

Skeletal muscle is all the muscles you voluntarily control, such as the muscles in your limbs, back, shoulders and so on. There are two other types, cardiac muscle is what the heart is formed of, whilst smooth muscle is your involuntary muscles – which includes muscles around your blood vessels, face and various parts of organs and other tissues.

Skeletal muscle is separated into two different groups, the blandly named type-1 and type-2. Type 1 muscle is effective at continued, sustained activity whereas type-2 muscle is effective at short, intense periods of activity. So, for example, you would predominantly use type-1 muscles for jogging, but type-2 muscles for sprinting.

Sirt-1 protects the type-1 muscles, but not the type-2 muscle, which is still broken down for energy. Therefore, holistic muscle mass drops when fasting, even though type-1 skeletal muscle mass increases.

Sirt-1 also influences how the muscles actually work. Sirt-1 is produced by the muscle cells, but the ability to produce Sirt-1 decreases as the muscle ages. As a result, muscle is harder to build as you age and doesn't grow as fast in response to exercise. A lack of sirt-1 also causes the muscles to become tired quicker and gradually decline over time.

When you start to consider these effects of Sirt-1, you can start to form a picture about why fasting helps keep the body supple. Fasting releases Sirt-1, which in turn helps skeletal muscle grow and stay in good shape. Sirt-1 is also released by consuming sirtuin activators, giving the Sirtfood diet its muscle retaining power.

On Aging

The old-age population covers nearly 55% of the total population on earth. The old-age population generally has people more than 50 years old. It is also called the geriatric population. Old age is a period of life in which many organs and organ systems begin to decline in their functional capacities. A balanced diet, like the sirtfood diet, can help in delaying the aging process.

Following are some benefits of using the sirtfood diet in old age:

- It helps in delaying the aging process

- The polyphenols are known as anti-aging mediators who are present in massive amounts in the sirtfood diet.

- The sirtfood diet helps in lowering cholesterol levels, and thus, a significant reduction of risk factors associated with heart attacks and stroke can be seen.

- This diet helps in proper turgor of skin to reduce freckles and pressure sores.

- Vitamin C rich diet helps in boosting immunity during the old age.

- Reproductive capacities can be maintained by following the sirtfood diet in old age.

- Risks of osteoporosis and other calcium-related disorders can be prevented.

- The sirtfood diet helps in keeping you moving during old age.

- Vital capacities of heart, lungs and other vital organs can be preserved by following the sirtfood diet

- It keeps your gut healthy, and thus constipation and infections can be prevented.

Insulin

Another claim expounded is that the Sirtfood diet also helps control diabetes. Some studies have found an association between Sirt-1 and the volume of insulin that can be released into the body. If you are familiar with the science behind diabetes, you may be aware that insulin is the hormone primarily responsible for controlling the levels of sugar in the blood. Therefore by increasing the amount of insulin that can be released, sirt-1 can theoretically help tackle diabetes by causing higher amounts of blood sugar to be converted into fat.

CHAPTER 8:

Weight Loss

What is the first thing that comes to mind when you hear the word "diet"? Most people think of losing weight and food restriction. There are hundreds of methods to lose weight in the market, and if you have a constant battle with your weight, you have probably heard of the majority, we go on a new diet per week - or almost

We know that diets, such as 5: 2 or "fasting" activate the so-called "skinny gene", it works for some people, but in the end, if you are hungry, you will probably be in a bad mood and even suffer attention deficit that is not only a problem at work, but it can be dangerous. Personally, I have nothing against 5: 2 that can be very useful for people who have a hard time with a daily caloric restriction for a sustained period of time. Very restrictive diets have a very high abandonment rate, the dieter gets fed up easily and leaves.

The name already reveals what the diet is basically focused on: all those foods which stimulate the fat-burning enzyme sirtuin and reduce the extra pounds are called sirt foods.

The scientific knowledge that certain plant compounds induce the function of the body's own sirtuins, as well as fasting, is the basis of the sirt food diet. For instance, Aidan Goggins and Glen Metten, the nutritionists and writers of the same-named diet bestseller, are persuaded that a diet based on the Sirtuin concept leads not only to a dream figure but also to enjoy. So long as you targeted blend the appropriate foods and outsource your metabolism in that way.

Examples of the secondary plant substances known to be sirtuin activators are allicin, which gives the garlic its traditional aroma, capsaicin, found mainly in chilies, or curcumin, to which the turmeric owes its yellow color.

Sirtfoods not only effectively improve fat burning, but they also protect the organism from cell damage, heart or cancer diseases and delay the overall aging cycle. Sirtuins also avoid traditional cravings, encourage muscle building and cellular health and reinforce the immune system. What makes a sirtuin diet so much easier: Sirtfoods are not rare or bland at all. Those are daily foods, particularly fruits and vegetables. Red wine and chocolate are allowed, by the way, too.

The Role of Sirtuins in the Body

In light of numerous studies, sirtuins play an extremely important role in the functioning of the body. They are credited with participating in many cellular processes. They participate in post-translational modification of other proteins, silencing gene transcription, activating repair mechanisms, as well as in regulating many metabolic processes, including lipid-carbohydrate metabolism and apoptosis. Their participation in stimulating growth and promoting cell survival is also suggested.

They gained popularity relatively recently when the discovery was made, showing a significant impact of their activity on aging processes. Research results have shown that short-term caloric restriction (CR) restriction in humans, and long-term in animals, causes changes in the intensity of metabolism, in the functioning of the endocrine and sympathetic nervous system, as well as affects the expression of genes in muscle cells, heart and the brain. The combination of all these changes in the body can, as a consequence, affect the delay in aging. This effect does not occur when the body is damaged or inactive genes encoding sirtuins. The role of Sir2 proteins in delaying aging is also associated with the reduction of reactive oxygen species (ROS) in cells, inhibition of apoptosis, as well as stimulating DNA damage repair.

The influence of sirtuins on a number of processes occurring in cells caused that they began to be seen as the possibility of therapeutic use. Research on their expression during many diseases suggests that regulation of their activity may bring results in the treatment of some metabolic, neurodegenerative, and cardiovascular diseases.

Sir2 proteins are found in almost all living organisms, but, regardless of their origin, are characterized by a high degree of similarity in the amino acid sequence. They belong to the family of histone deacetylases, catalyzing two reactions dependent on NAD + hydrolysis: deacetylation and mono - ADP - ribosylation. In light of numerous studies, sirtuins play an extremely important role in the functioning of the body. Depending on their location, in the cell nucleus, mitochondria or cytoplasm, they perform a number of functions. Sir2 proteins are attributed to participation in many cellular processes, such as post-translational protein modification, gene silencing, activation of DNA repair mechanisms, as well as the regulation of many metabolic processes.

Sir2 proteins are found in almost all living organisms, but, regardless of their origin, are characterized by a high degree of similarity in the amino acid sequence. They are able to catalyze two types of reactions, deacetylation and mono - ADP - ribosylation, but it is enough to play an important role in the proper functioning of the body. In mammals, their activity is associated with increased resistance to stress factors and many metabolic pathways, such as adipogenesis, angiogenesis, gluconeogenesis and maintaining proper insulin and glucose levels in the blood. The ability of sirtuins to regulate metabolism, DNA repair processes, apoptosis and lowering of ROS levels in cells gives these little-known enzymes a great deal of importance.

Current research is aimed at expanding knowledge about the detailed mechanisms of sirtuins and their possible use in the treatment of metabolic diseases and age-related diseases. Activation or inhibition of their activity is seen as the possibility of creating selective and effective therapy methods.

In addition, sirtuins play an important role in aging processes and regulating life expectancy. Further research into the molecular basis of sirtuins may, perhaps, allow for the generation of new generation drugs that stop the progression of aging and allow for longer preservation of youth, health, and vitality.

Sirtuins also affect the metabolism of sugars and fats. They activate various transcription factors, e.g., FOXO1, which causes the expression of genes associated with gluconeogenesis. It has also been shown that SIRT proteins interact directly with various enzymes of metabolic pathways, e.g., phosphoenolpyruvate carboxykinase, thus increasing its activity. Many studies have shown that in the case of sugar metabolism, these proteins promote gluconeogenesis while slowing down glycolysis (by activating appropriate transcription factors), and in the case of fat metabolism, they initiate β-oxidation and inhibit lipogenesis and adipocytogenesis.

Role of Sirtuins and Metabolic Activities

Following the discovery in 2003, Sirt's food was enthusiastic. Studies show that the effects of calorie restriction are not imitated simply by these foods. They also serve as super-regulators for the entire metabolism, burning fat, rising muscle weight, and enhancing cell santé. Scientific work was closely linked to the century's most significant nutritional discovery. Sadly, there was a mistake: in an attempt to turn sirt food into a miracle pill, the pharmaceutical industry invested hundreds of millions of pounds, and the diet had taken a back seat. We have no pharmaceutical approach to concentrate the advantages of those complex plant-origin nutrients into one single medicine (so far without any results). It seems more prudent to take the most advantage of the natural ingredients, the nutrients in the foods we consume, instead of waiting for pharmaceutical companies to transform into a miracle drug (which does not work anyway). This is the basis of our pilot experiments in order to create and observe a diet that contains the richest sources of Sirt food.

CHAPTER 9:

Sirtfood Diet and Workout

Sirtfood diet is more like an alternate way of living as compared to any ordinary diet plan. For most people, losing weight or just maintaining a normal body weight might turn out to be a difficult job. However, seeking the help of sirtfood diet can help in losing weight without any kind of extra effort. But, can you combine a sirtfood diet with your daily workout routine? Well, the answer is yes. You can continue with your workout routine while following the sirtdiet.

It has been found that about 750 million adults are currently suffering from the problems of obesity in the entire world. So, it is very important to find some healthy eating habits along with exercise routines so that you can deal with all such problems easily. You will need to find something that will not be taking you away from the opportunity of enjoying life and will not require you to keep working out the entire day. All of these requirements can be handled single-handedly by sirtdiet. The main idea of this diet is that certain food items will activate the sirtuins that generally gets activated with the help of fasting and working out.

During the two phases of the diet, it is recommended just to pause your workout routine or lower the intensity. The main reason behind this is that the diet focuses on calorie restriction. When you reduce all the physical activities, the body will find it a lot easier to adapt itself to the changed calorie consumption. All that you will need to do is to listen to your body. If you are feeling fatigued or feeling tired, it will be better for you to stop working during the phases of the diet. You can give that time to be focused on the principles of the sirtdiet for leading a healthy life.

Working Out After the Phases of The Diet

You can definitely resume your old workout routine after you have successfully completed the diet phases. You will need to ensure that you consume enough protein in your diet to help in the recovery of the muscles. One of the unique aspects of sirtdiet is that you will not be losing your muscle mass. The diet will aid in losing excess fat only. So, even athletes can opt for this diet but make sure that you are gentle on yourself during the first few days of the diet until your body adapts itself completely to the changed routine. In case you exercise at moderate intensity, you can continue with your exercise routine during the diet as well. Everything will depend on you, the extent to which you can push yourself to bring the required alteration in your life. You will need to manage your fitness routine in accordance with the diet plan.

Working Out and Its Importance

Exercising is all about various movements that can help in burning calories and make the muscles work at a faster rate. If you are trying to start with daily exercise, you can opt for walking, jogging, running, dancing, swimming, and others. When you start exercising along with a proper diet plan, it can impart several benefits to your body and health. You will be able to shed more kilos with the help of moderate exercising along with sirtdiet.

It Can Help In Losing Weight

The primary goal of the sirtfood diet is to shed the extra pounds from the body. When you make yourself inactive or opt for very few activities, it will result in weight gain and obesity. For getting proper knowledge about the effect of working out on weight loss, you will need first to understand the connection between exercise and expenditure of energy. You can spend all your energy in three ways: digestion, maintenance of physical functions like heartbeat and breathing, and exercising. When you start with the sirtfood diet, the consumption of calories will be restricted and that will result in lowering down the metabolic rate of the body. This can lead to a delay in weight loss. On the contrary, as you start exercising along with the diet, you can improve the rate of metabolism that will ultimately be burning down calories. So, in this way, you can lose more weight with no effect on muscle mass.

If you want to start with exercising, start by combining resistance training along with aerobic exercises. It can intensify the whole process, and you will be able to build up muscle mass as well. So, you will need to start with moderate exercises after you complete both the phases of the diet.

It Can Make You Feel Happy

It has been found that exercising can help in improving the quality of your mood. In fact, exercise can easily deal with stress, anxiety, and extreme depression. When you start with the diet, the body will go into a state of shock during the initial days. This is because there will be a restriction of calories. If you opt for moderate exercising along with the diet, your body will find it easier to deal with the stress of this nature. As you exercise, it makes certain changes in the brain that can help in dealing with stress and anxiety. Also, exercising can help in improving the brain sensitivity for certain hormones like serotonin and norepinephrine that are responsible for relieving depression.

Exercising helps in improving the production of endorphins that can are responsible for dealing with pain and positive feelings. Exercise has shown a positive impact on all those people who suffer from extreme anxiety. With the help of exercise, you can make yourself aware of the mental state. When you lower down the calorie consumption during the initial stages of the diet, you can develop a very disturbing mood. You can start exercising for keeping your mood under proper control. Moreover, you will be able to bring about better changes as you opt for moderate exercise along with the diet.

CHAPTER 10:

The Right Mindset to Lose Weight

Drink healthy

Because it is useless to eat the right foods if you do not have the appropriate patent.

It is estimated that people swallow an additional 200 calories per day, just in their drinks (hello? Sodas?!). So we get used to drinking water, herbal teas, tea, sugar-free coffee, and we forget sodas, yes, even with fake sugar that will only preserve your unreasonable taste for the sugar.

Eat a variety

Diets are repetitive and lead straight on the road to boredom? So the key is variety.

Be curious, vary the pleasures, the food, and the colors. Color your plate of fruits and vegetables which are excellent antioxidants, consume" good fats seeds and oilseeds such as almonds, whole grains. "

Maintain physical activity

An active lifestyle is essential for health (and not only at the heart level). The World Health Organization recommends that you walk at least 6,000 steps per day in a dynamic manner, in particular to regulate the blood sugar level.

If you have a job where you mainly sit, then discipline yourself: 15 min of exercise in the morning, get up and go for a walk every 2 hours during the day, walk before going home or walk the dog, and practice a sport ideally twice a week.

Say stop to the yo-yo effect

We know it, when we want to lose weight, it's always the same thing: we make efforts then we crack, and bim! It is left for new efforts etc. etc.

Studies show that the people who lose weight the most sustainably are those who have managed to adopt a healthy diet by starting with small changes. So, instead of giving up on chocolate completely, make sure you don't overuse other things so that you can preserve that little treat. Also learn to limit yourself to a few squares of dark chocolate rather than devouring a plate of super sweet milk chocolate.

Getting into running

Running is one of those sports that promote weight loss, even if you run slowly. What if you signed up for a race to motivate yourself?

Eat more often at home

Unless you are super strong and can resist multiple temptations, when you go out to dinner, it is rare to choose the healthiest dishes, to ignore the wine and to deprive of dessert. In addition, the quality of the food we eat is absolutely not guaranteed and we quickly eat too sweet, too fatty & too salty.

Likewise when you are invited, you must learn not to nibble as an aperitif, to drink water when necessary. Not easy! So the best way to put the slider for better eating back in the center, is at least to eat most often at home, in order to prepare your menu knowingly. And if you don't want to let go of your social life: invite!

As for meals during the work week, prepare two parts when you cook something good, so take the leftovers to warm up at the office.

Controlled portions

The idea here is not to frustrate you by forcing you to eat less, but rather to know how to identify your needs so as not to eat more than reason. Because the more we eat, the more our stomach distends and prepares to receive more and more food.

It is often recommended during a full meal to fill your plate: from a third to a half of raw and cooked vegetables, and if you like legumes, make sure to mix with green vegetables, tomatoes, carrots ... Then, a third of complex carbohydrates such as wholegrain rice, sweet potato, and a third of protein (and not necessarily meat).

We can then modulate with legumes instead of animal proteins, wakame algae instead of green beans, etc.

A different social life

Rather than always meeting your friends around a cocktail or a raclette, offer them other activities. A bike ride with a picnic, a fitness session with friends, an exhibition with guided tour, a tea tasting workshop.

CHAPTER 11:

Step By Step Sirtfood Diet

Step 1: Heavy Weight Loss

Phase 1 of the diet is the one that produces the greatest results. Over the course of seven days, you will follow a simple method in order to lose 3.5 kg.

During the first three days, the intake of calories will have to be limited to one thousand per day at most. Basically, you can have three green juices and a solid meal, all based on Sirt foods. From day 4 to 7, the daily calories will become fifteen hundred. Every day you will eat two green juices and two solid Sirt meals. By the end of the seven days, you should have lost, on average, 3.5 kilos.

Monday: 3 green juices

- Breakfast: water + tea or espresso + a cup of green juice;

- Lunch: green juice

- Snack: a square of dark chocolate;

- Dinner: Sirt meal

- After dinner: a square of dark chocolate.

Drink the juices at three distinct times of the day (for example, in the morning as soon as you wake up, mid-morning and mid-afternoon) and choose a normal or vegan dish

Tuesday: 3 green juices

- Breakfast: water + tea or espresso + a cup of green juice

- Lunch: 2 green juices before dinner;

- Snack: a square of dark chocolate;

- Dinner: Sirt meal

- After dinner: a square of dark chocolate.

Welcome to day 2 of the Sirtfood Diet. The formula is identical to that of the first day, and the only thing that changes is the solid meal. Today you will also have dark chocolate, and the same goes for tomorrow. This food is so wonderful that we don't need an excuse to eat it.

On day 2, capers are also included in the menu. Despite what many may think, they are not fruits, but buds that grow in Mediterranean countries and are picked by hand. They are fantastic Sirt foods because they are very rich in the nutrients kaempferol and quercetin. From the point of view of flavor, they are tiny concentrates of taste. If you've never used them, don't feel intimidated. You will see, they will taste amazingly if combined with the right ingredients, and they will give an unmistakable and inimitable aroma to your dishes.

On the second day, you will intake: 3 green Sirt juices and one solid meal (normal or vegan).

Drink the juices at three distinct times of the day (for example, when you wake up in the morning, mid-morning and mid-afternoon) and choose either a normal or the vegan dish.

Wednesday: 3 green juices

- Breakfast: water + tea or espresso + a cup of green juice

- Lunch: 2 green juices before dinner;

- Snack: a square of dark chocolate;

- Dinner: Sirt meal

- After dinner: a square of dark chocolate.

You are now on the third day, and even if the format is once again identical to that of days 1 and 2, so the time has come to flavor everything with a fundamental ingredient. For thousands of years, chili has been a fundamental element of the gastronomic experiences of the whole world.

If you are not a big expert of chili, we recommend the Bird's Eye (sometimes called Thai chili), because it is the best for sirtuins.

This is the last day you will consume three green juices a day; tomorrow, you will switch to two. We, therefore, take this opportunity to browse other drinks that you can have during the diet. We all know that green tea is good for health, and water is naturally very good, but what about coffee? More than half of people drink at least one coffee a day, but always with a trace of guilt because some say that it is a vice and an unhealthy habit. This is absolutely untrue; studies show that coffee is a real treasure trove of beneficial plant substances. That's why coffee drinkers run the least risk of getting diabetes, certain forms of cancer, and neurodegenerative diseases. Furthermore, not only is coffee, not a toxin, it protects the liver and makes it even healthier!

On the third day, you will intake 3 green Sirt juices and 1 one solid meal (normal or vegan, see below).

Drink the juices at three distinct times of the day (for example, in the morning as soon as you wake up, mid-morning and mid-afternoon) and choose a normal or vegan dish.

Thursday: 3 green juices

- Breakfast: water + tea or espresso + a cup of green juice;

- Lunch: Sirt food;

- Snack: 1 green juice before dinner

- Dinner: Sirt food

The fourth day of the Sirtfood Diet has arrived, and you are halfway through your journey to a leaner and healthier body. The big change from the preceding three days is that you will only drink two juices instead of three and that you will have two solid meals instead of one. This means that on the fourth day and the upcoming ones, you will have two green juices and two solid meals, all delicious and rich in Sirt foods. The inclusion of Medjoul dates in a list of foods that promote weight loss and good health may seem surprising. Especially when you think they contain 66 percent sugar.

Today we will also integrate chicory into meals. Like with onion, red chicory is better in this case too, but endive, its close relative, is also a Sirt food. If you are looking for ideas on the use of these salads, combine them with other varieties and season them with olive oil: they will give a pungent flavor to milder leaves.

On the fourth day, you will intake: 2 green Sirt juices, 2 solid meals (normal or vegan)

Drink the juices at different times of the day (for example the first in the morning as soon as you wake up or in the middle of the morning, the second in the middle of the afternoon) and choose normal or vegan dishes.

Friday: 2 green juices

Breakfast: water + tea or espresso + a cup of green juice

- Lunch: Sirt food

- Snack: a green juice before dinner;

- Dinner: Sirt food

You have reached the fifth day, and the time has come to add fruits. Due to its high sugar content, fruits have been the subject of bad publicity. This does not apply to berries. Strawberries have a very low sugar content: one teaspoon per 100 grams. They also have an excellent effect on how the body processes simple sugars.

On the fifth day, you will intake 2 green Sirt juices and 2 solid meals (normal or vegan).

Drink the juices at different times of the day (for example the first in the morning as soon as you wake up or in the middle of the morning, the second in the middle of the afternoon) and choose normal or vegan dishes.

Saturday: 2 green juices

- Breakfast: water + tea or espresso + a cup of green juice

- Lunch: Sirt food

- Snack: a green juice before dinner;

- Dinner: Sirt food

On the sixth day, you will assume 2 green Sirt juices and 2 solid meals (normal or vegan).

Drink the juices at different times of the day (for example, the first in the morning as soon as you wake up or in the middle of the morning, the second in the middle of the afternoon) and choose normal or vegan dishes.

Sunday: 2 green juices

- Breakfast: a bowl of Sirt Muesli + a cup of green juice

- Lunch: Sirt food

- Snack: a cup of green juice;

- dinner: Sirt food

The seventh day is the last of phase 1 of the diet. Instead of considering it as an end, see it as a beginning, because you are about to embark on a new life, in which Sirt foods will play a central role in your nutrition. Today's menu is a perfect example of how easy it is to integrate them in abundance into your daily diet. Just take your favorite dishes and, with a pinch of creativity, you will turn them into a Sirt banquet.

On the seventh day, you will assume 2 green Sirt juices; 2 solid meals (normal or vegan).

Drink the juices at different times of the day (for example the first in the morning as soon as you wake up or in the middle of the morning, the second in the middle of the afternoon) and choose normal or vegan dishes.

During the second phase, there are no calorie restrictions but indications on which Sirt foods must be eaten to consolidate weight loss and not run the risk of getting the lost kilograms back.

Step 2: Maintenance

Congratulations on completing Sirtfood Diet Step 1! You will already see amazing results with a weight loss and not only look slimmer and more toned but also feel revitalized and re-energized. So, now what?

Having seen these often-remarkable transformations firsthand ourselves, we know how much you are going to want to see even better results, not just preserve all those beets. Sirtfoods are, after all, designed to eat for life. The problem is how you adapt what you did in Phase 1 into your regular dietary routine. That's precisely what prompted us to develop a fourteen-day maintenance plan designed to help you make the transition from Phase 1 to your more usual dietary routine, thus helping to maintain and expand the Sirtfood Diet's benevolence.

What to Expect

You should maintain your weight-loss results during Phase 2, and continue to lose weight gradually.

Also, the one striking thing we've found with the Sirtfood Diet is that most or all of the weight people lose is from fat and that many put some muscle in. So we would like to remind you again not to measure your success solely on the scale by the numbers. Look in the mirror to see if you look leaner and more toned, see how your clothes are tingling, and lap up the compliments you're going to get from others.

Also remember that as the weight loss continues, so will the health beets increase. By following the 14-day maintenance plan, you are starting to lay the foundations for a lifelong health future.

How to Follow Phase 2

The key to success in this process is keeping your diet filled with Sirtfoods. To make it as simple as possible, we have prepared a seven-day menu plan for you to follow, including delicious family-friendly recipes, filled with Sirtfoods every day to the rafters (although see page 149 for children's advice). All you need to do is repeat the Seven Day Plan twice to complete Phase 2's fourteen days.

On each of the fourteen days, your diet will consist of:

- 3 x balanced sirtfood-rich meals
- 1 x sirtfood green juice
- 1 to 2 x optional snacks Sirtfood bite snacks

Once again, when you have to consume these, there are no rigid rules. Be flexible throughout your day, and t them. Two simple thumb rules are:

- Have your green juice either in the morning, at least 30 minutes before breakfast, or in the middle of the morning.
- Do your hardest to eat your dinner by 7 p.m.

Portion Sizes

During Phase 2, our attention is not on calorie counting. For the average person, this is not a practical approach or even a successful one over the long term. Alternatively, we concentrate on small servings, really well-balanced meals, and, most importantly, filling up on Sirtfoods so that you can continue to enjoy their fat burning and health-promoting effects.

What to Drink

In phase 2, you can need to have one green juice per day. This is to keep you top with high Sirtfoods levels.

Just as in Phase 1, during Phase 2, you can freely ingest other fluids. Our favorite beverages include remaining plain water, homemade flavored beer, coffee, and green tea. If black or white tea is your predilection, feel free to enjoy it. The same goes for herbal teas. The best news is that during Phase 2, you can enjoy the occasional glass of red wine. Due to its content of sirtuin-activating polyphenols, particularly resveratrol and piceatannol, red wine is a sirtfood which makes it by far the best choice of alcoholic beverage. But, with alcohol itself having adverse effects on our fat cells, moderation is still best, and we recommend limiting your intake to one glass of red wine with a meal for two or three days a week throughout Phase 2.

Returning To Three Meals

You ate only one or two meals a day during Phase 1, which gave you plenty of leisure time to eat your meals. As we are now returning to a more usual schedule and the time-tested practice of three meals a day, thinking about breakfast is a good time.

Eating a healthy breakfast sets us ready for the day, raising our levels of strength and focus. Eating earlier keeps our blood sugar and fat levels in check, in terms of our metabolism. That breakfast is a good thing is borne out by several studies, typically showing that people who eat breakfast regularly are less likely to overweight.

That is because of our internal body clocks. Our bodies are expecting us to eat early in anticipation of when we will be most busy and need food. Yet as many as a thirds of us will miss breakfasts on any given day. It's a classic symptom of our busy modern life, and the impression is there's simply not enough time to eat well. But as you will see, nothing could be further from the truth with the nifty breakfasts that we have laid out here for you. Whether it's the Sirtfood smoothie that can be drunk on the go, the premade Sirt muesli or the fast and easy Sirtfood scrambled eggs/tofu, finding those extra few minutes in the morning, will yield rewards not only for your day but for your weight and health over the longer term.

With Sirtfoods working to overcharge our energy levels, there's, even more, to gain from getting a hit from them early in the morning to start your day. This is done not only by eating a Sirtfood-rich meal but also by consuming the green juice, which we suggest you have either first thing in the morning — at least thirty minutes before a meal — or mid-morning.

"Sirtifying" Your Meals

We've noticed that inclusion, not exclusion are the only healthy diet. But real success goes beyond this — the food has to be consistent with living in modern times. Whether it's the ease of meeting our hectic life's demands or fitting in with our position as the bon vivant at dinner parties, the way we eat should be trouble-free. You will enjoy your svelte figure and radiant glow, rather than thinking about the demands and restrictions of kooky foods.

What makes Sirtfoods so fantastic is that they are very available, familiar, and comfortable to include in your diet. Here, as you cross the gap between step 1 and routine eating, you can lay the groundwork for a new, enhanced lifelong eating strategy.

CHAPTER 12:

Post Diet

Getting more fit is sometimes very strenuous. However, dieters are likewise confronted with the way that situation is anything but favorable for them for long haul achievement. Analysts gauge that just around 20 percent of dieters keep up weight loss after a diet. Is it accurate to say that you will be one of them?

Step by Step Instructions to Maintain Weight Loss After A Diet

To build your odds of weight support after a diet, plan for a transitional phase after you arrive at your objective weight. During this time, make moderate changes following your way of life and watch the consequences for the scale.

This transitional phase is additionally a decent time to recognize the eating propensities and exercise designs that you learned while dieting so you can keep up as long as possible. If you transform healthy diet propensities into a healthy way of life propensities, you're probably going to forestall weight recapture. Specialists have discovered that dieters who keep the weight off for good are the individuals who keep on keeping up a low-fat diet with a lot of foods from the ground.

Ten Habits to Help You Maintain Your Weight

The ten propensities beneath will assist you with moving from the first phase, through the maintenance phase, lastly into the support phase, where your weight stays stable. To improve your odds of perpetual weight-loss achievement, attempt to fuse these ten propensities into your way of life as you travel through all phases of the dieting venture.

Moderate Weight Loss Works Best

Doctors suggest that dieters lose close to one to two pounds every week. This moderate methodology assists patients with maintaining a strategic distance from wellbeing dangers related to extraordinary weight loss. It likewise permits the dieter to learn new eating propensities that will ensure their weight loss over the long haul. Segment control, healthy eating, ordinary exercise, and perusing dietary names are key aptitudes that you'll ace if you pick the more slow way to deal with weight loss.

Make Moderate Progress Out of The Dieting Stage

When you arrive at your objective weight, the most exceedingly terrible thing you can do is to continue your old eating propensities. Recollect that those are the eating propensities that caused the weight gain in any case. It is sensible to step by step increment caloric admission, yet specialists, for the most part, propose including just 200 calories for each week until your weight balances out.

. Stay Associated with Your Wellsprings of Help

Similar individuals who bolstered you in the dieting procedure will assist you with keeping up your weight loss. They are in the best situation to regard the size of your achievement and give you a delicate update if you forget about your prosperity. Speak with them and give them consent to offer an aware direction if necessary.

Continue to Challenge Yourself with New Objectives

Since you've aced probably the hardest test you'll ever confront, remain on your toes by defining another objective. It doesn't need to be identified with weight loss. Accomplishing both present moment and long haul objectives will assist you with keeping your certainty level high.

Remain Taught

Take healthy-cooking classes, go to wellbeing workshops, and take an interest in wellness fairs. Encircle yourself with tokens of what carrying on with a healthy life truly implies. You may likewise need to remain included on the web.

Become A Coach

Probably an ideal approach to remain instructed is to show your weight-loss aptitudes to an amateur. By turning into a coach, you'll be required to keep steady over new research and patterns.

Exercise

An investigation into changeless weight loss uncovers that activity is probably the best indicator of long haul achievement. Thirty to an hour of moderate exercise each day will keep both your body and psyche healthy.

Eat Breakfast

Studies have additionally discovered that individuals who eat breakfast are progressively effective at keeping the pounds under control. Ensure that your breakfast incorporates entire grains and a lean wellspring of protein.

Weigh Yourself

Use a scale once a week to monitor your weight. Studies show that checking it all the time is a training shared by individuals who effectively keep their weight off.

Keep Standard Meetings with Your Social Insurance Group

Your human services supplier or enlisted dietician will have the option to quantify your muscle to fat ratio or assess your BMI to ensure that your numbers remain healthy. They will have the option to address medical problems that emerge when your body shape changes.

CHAPTER 13:

Breakfast Recipes

Matcha Green Juice

Preparation Time: 10 minutes

Cooking time: 0 minutes

Servings: 2

Ingredients:

5 ounces fresh kale - 2 ounces fresh arugula

¼ cup fresh parsley - 4 celery stalks

1 green apple, cored and chopped - 1 (1-inch) piece fresh ginger, peeled

1 lemon, peeled - ½ teaspoon matcha green tea

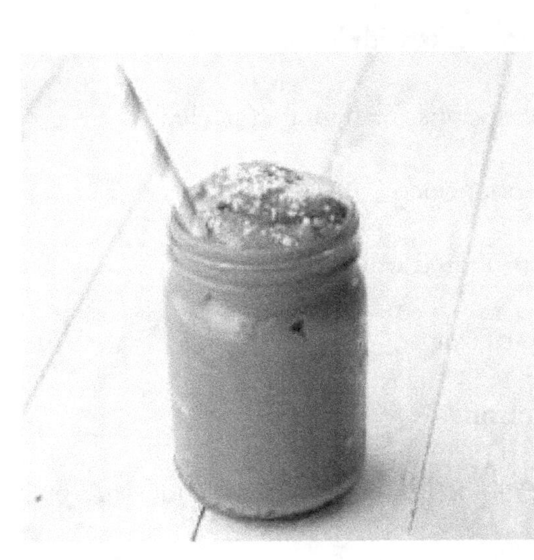

Directions:

Add all ingredients into a juicer and extract the juice according to the manufacturer's method.

Pour into 2 glasses and serve immediately.

Nutrition:

Calories 113 Fat 0.6 g

Carbs 26.71 g Protein 3.8 g

Celery Juice

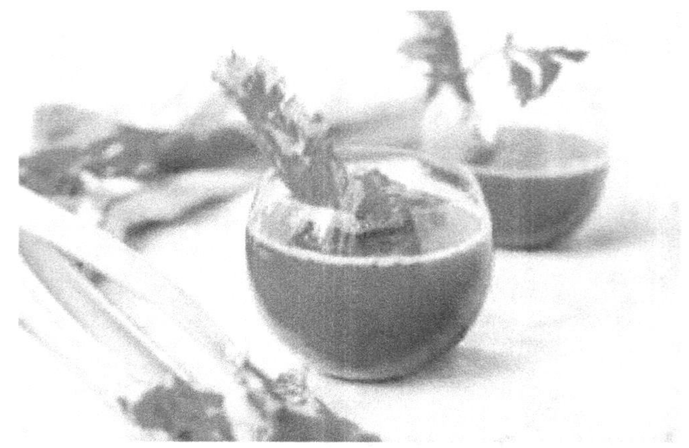

Preparation Time: 10 minutes

Cooking time: 0 minutes

Servings: 2

Ingredients:

8 celery stalks with leaves

2 tablespoons fresh ginger, peeled

1 lemon, peeled

½ cup filtered water

Pinch of salt

Directions:

Place all the ingredients in a blender and pulse until well combined.

Through a fine mesh strainer, strain the juice and transfer into 2 glasses.

Serve immediately.

Nutrition:

Calories 32

Fat 0.5 g

Carbs 6.5 g

Protein 1 g

Kale & Orange Juice

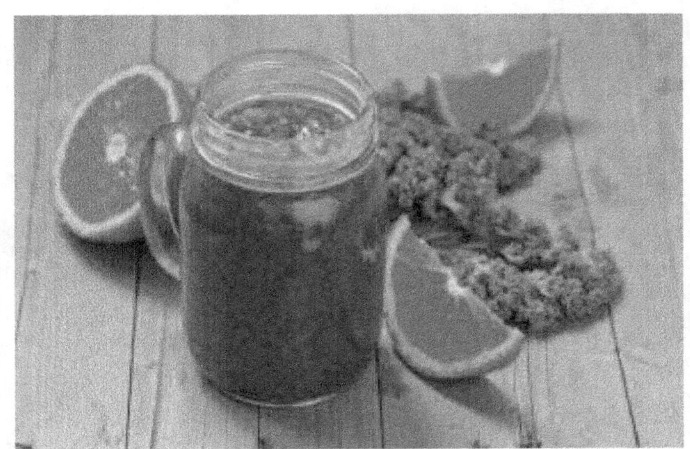

Preparation Time: 10 minutes

Cooking time: 0 minutes

Servings: 2

Ingredients:

5 large oranges, peeled and sectioned

2 bunches fresh kale

Directions:

Add all ingredients into a juicer and extract the juice according to the manufacturer's method.

Pour into 2 glasses and serve immediately.

Nutrition:

Calories 315

Fat 0.6 g

Carbs 75.1 g

Protein 10.3 g

Kale Scramble

Preparation Time: 10 minutes

Cooking time: 6 minutes

Servings: 2

Ingredients:

4 eggs

⅛ teaspoon ground turmeric

Salt and ground black pepper, to taste

1 tablespoon water

2 teaspoons olive oil

1 cup of fresh kale, (tough ribs removed and chopped

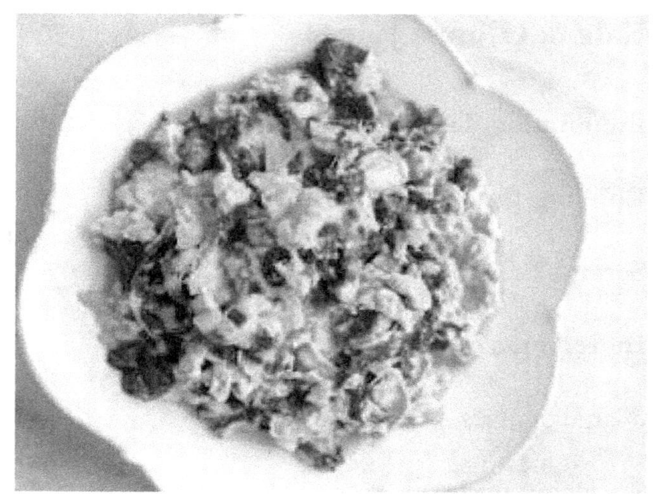

Directions:

In a bowl, add the eggs, turmeric, salt, black pepper, and water and with a whisk, beat until foamy.

In a wok, heat the oil over medium heat.

Add the egg mixture and stir to combine.

Immediately, reduce the heat to medium-low and cook for about 1–2 minutes, stirring frequently.

Stir in the kale and cook for about 3–4 minutes, stirring frequently.

Remove from the heat and serve immediately.

Nutrition:

Calories 183 Fat 13.4 g Carbs 4.3 g   Protein 12.1 g

Buckwheat Porridge

Preparation Time: 10 minutes

Cooking time: 15 minutes

Servings: 2

Ingredients:

1 cup buckwheat, rinsed

1 cup unsweetened almond milk

1 cup water

½ teaspoon ground cinnamon

½ teaspoon vanilla extract

1–2 tablespoons raw honey

¼ cup fresh blueberries

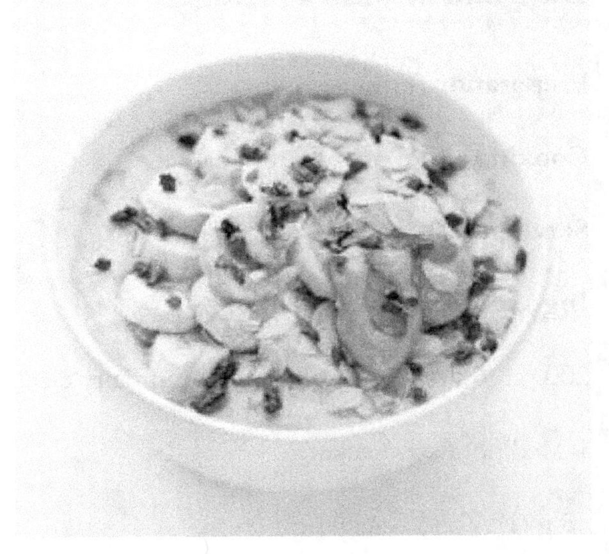

Directions:

In a pan, add all the ingredients (except honey and blueberries) over medium-high heat and bring to a boil. Now, reduce the heat to low and simmer, covered for about 10 minutes.

Stir in the honey and remove from the heat. Set aside, covered, for about 5 minutes.

With a fork, fluff the mixture, and transfer into serving bowls.

Top with blueberries and serve.

Nutrition:

Calories 358 Fat 4.7 g Carbs 3.7 g   Protein 12 g

Date and Walnut Porridge

Preparation Time: 55 minutes

Cooking time: 30 minutes

Servings: 2

Ingredients:

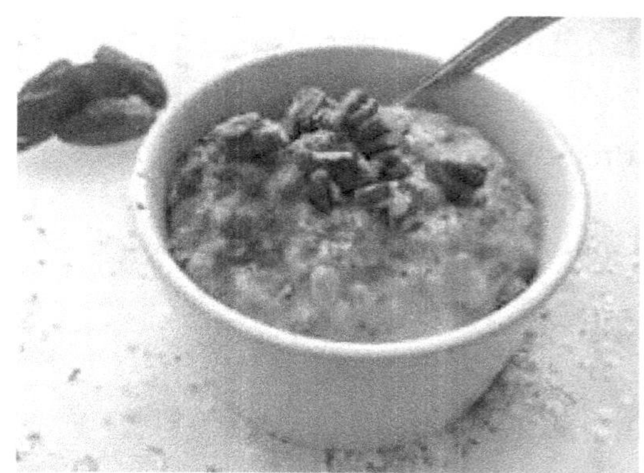

200 ml (6 ½ fl. oz.) Milk or without dairy elective

1 Medjool date, hacked

35 g (1 ¼ oz.) Buckwheat chips

1 tsp. Pecan spread or four cleaved pecan parts

50 g (1 ⅝ oz.) Strawberries, hulled

Directions:

Spot the milk and time in a dish, heat tenderly, at that point include the buckwheat chips and cook until the porridge is your ideal consistency.

Mix in the pecan margarine or pecans, top with the strawberries and serve.

Nutrition:

Calories: 66 kcal

Protein: 1.08 g

Fat: 1.07 g

Carbohydrates: 14.56 g

CHAPTER 14:

Lunch Recipes

Shrimp & Arugula Soup

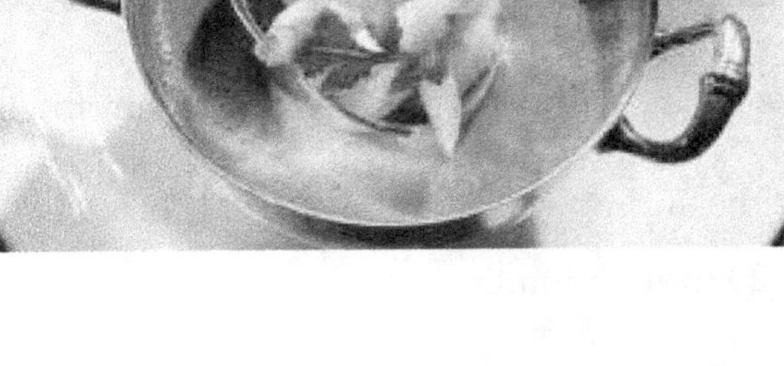

Preparation Time: 5 minutes

Cooking Time: 30 minutes

Servings: 3

Ingredients:

10 medium sized shrimp or 5 large prawns, cleaned, deshelled and deveined

1 small red onion, sliced very thinly

1 cup arugula

1 cup baby kale

2 large celery stalks, sliced very thinly

5 sprigs of parsley, chopped

11 cloves of garlic, minced

5 cups of chicken or fish or vegetable stock

1 tbsp. extra virgin olive oil

Dash of sea salt

Dash of pepper

Directions:

Sauté the vegetables (not the kale or arugula just yet however), in a stock pot, on low heat for about 2 minutes so that they are still tender and still crunchy, but not cooked quite yet.

You will need to save the Cook time for the next step.

Add the salt and pepper.

Next, clean and chop the shrimp into bite-sized pieces that would be comfortable eating in a soup.

Then, add the shrimp to the pot, and sauté for 10 more minutes on medium-low heat.

Make sure the shrimp is cooked thoroughly and is not translucent.

When the shrimp seems to be cooked through, add the stock to the pot and cook on medium for about 20 more minutes.

Remove from heat and cool before serving.

Nutrition:

Calories: 450

Carbs: 32g

Fat: 27g

Protein: 23g

Chicken and Lentil Stew

Preparation Time: 10 minutes

Cooking Time: 40 minutes

Servings: 3

Ingredients:

4 chicken breasts, diced - ½ cup red lentils, rinsed

1 carrot, chopped - 1 small onion, chopped

1 garlic clove, chopped - 1 celery stalk, chopped - 1 small red pepper, chopped

1 can tomatoes, chopped

1 tbsp. paprika

1 tsp ginger, grated

3 tbsp. extra virgin olive oil

½ cup fresh parsley leaves, finely cut, to serve

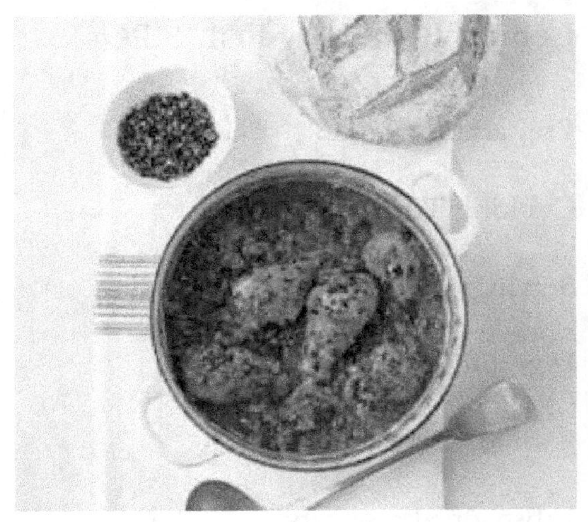

Directions:

Heat olive oil in a casserole and gently brown the chicken, stirring. Add in onions, garlic, celery, carrot, pepper, paprika and ginger. Cook, stirring constantly, for 2-3 minutes. Add in the lentils and tomatoes and bring to a boil.

Lower heat, cover, and simmer for 30 minutes, or until the lentils are tender and the chicken is cooked through. Serve sprinkled with fresh parsley.

Nutrition:

Calories: 311 Carbs: 36g Fat: 4g Protein: 32g

Lemon Rosemary Fish Fillets

Preparation Time: 10 minutes

Cooking Time: 25 minutes

Servings: 3

Ingredients:

4 white fish fillets

1 tbsp. dried rosemary

4 tbsp. breadcrumbs

2 tbsp. lemon zest

1 tsp garlic powder

2 tbsp. extra virgin olive oil

1 tsp salt

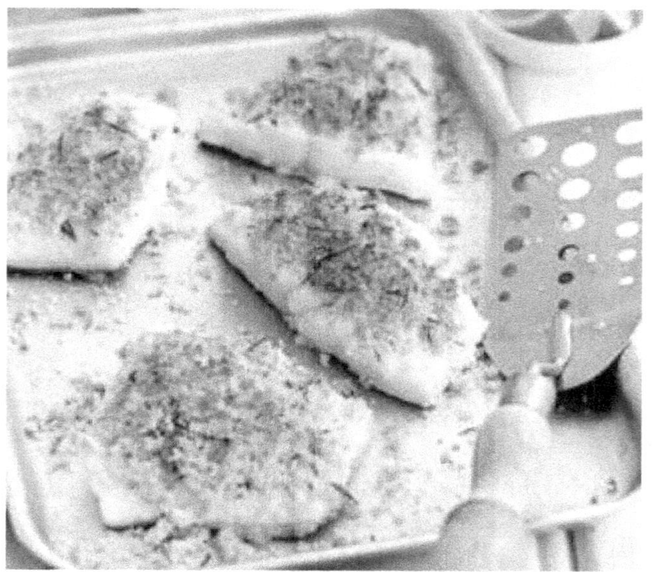

Directions:

Combine the rosemary, breadcrumbs, lemon zest, garlic powder and salt in a food processor and blend until well mixed. Add the fish fillets, skin-side up, on a lined baking tray.

Grill for 3-4 minutes. Turn the fish over and press a quarter of the breadcrumb mixture over the top of each fillet.

Drizzle with olive oil and grill for 4 min until the crust is golden and the fish is cooked through.

Serve with steamed spinach or baked potatoes.

Nutrition:

Calories: 100 Carbs: 0g Fat: 3g Protein: 17g

Healthy Chicken and Oat Soup

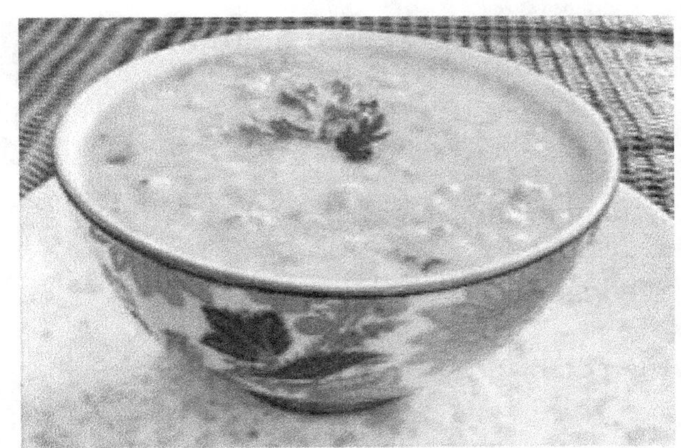

Preparation Time: 5 minutes

Cooking Time: 40 minutes

Servings: 3

Ingredients:

3 chicken breasts, diced

1 small onion, chopped - 3 garlic cloves - ½ cup quick-cooking oats

1 large carrot, chopped

1 red bell pepper, chopped

1 celery rib, chopped

1 tomato, diced

5 cups water

1 bay leaf

1 tsp salt

½ cup fresh parsley leaves, finely cut - Black pepper, to taste

Directions:

Place the chicken, bay leaf, celery, carrot, onion, red pepper, tomato and salt into a soup pot. Add in water and bring to the boil then reduce heat and simmer for 30 minutes. Discard the bay leaf, season with salt and pepper, add in the oats and parsley, simmer for 5 more minutes, and serve.

Nutrition:

Calories: 80 Carbs: 23g Fat: 2g Protein: 7g

Mediterranean Baked Salmon

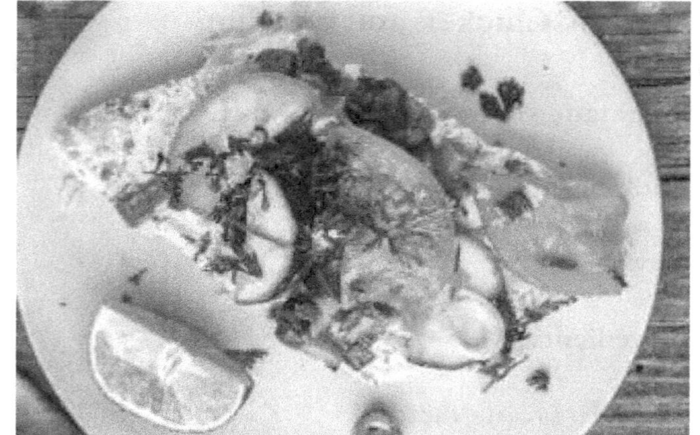

Preparation Time: 5 minutes

Cooking Time: 30 minutes

Servings: 3

Ingredients:

2 (6 oz.) boneless salmon fillets

1 tomato, thinly sliced

1 onion, thinly sliced

1 tbsp. capers

3 tbsp. olive oil

1 tsp dry oregano

3 tbsp. parmesan cheese

Salt and black pepper, to taste

Directions:

Preheat oven to 350°F.

Add salmon fillets in a baking dish, sprinkle with oregano, top with onion and tomato slices, drizzle with olive oil, and sprinkle with capers and parmesan cheese.

Cover the dish with foil and bake for 30 minutes, or until the fish flakes easily.

Nutrition:

Calories: 339 Carbs: 5g Fat: 18g Protein: 37g

Chicken with Broccoli & Mushrooms

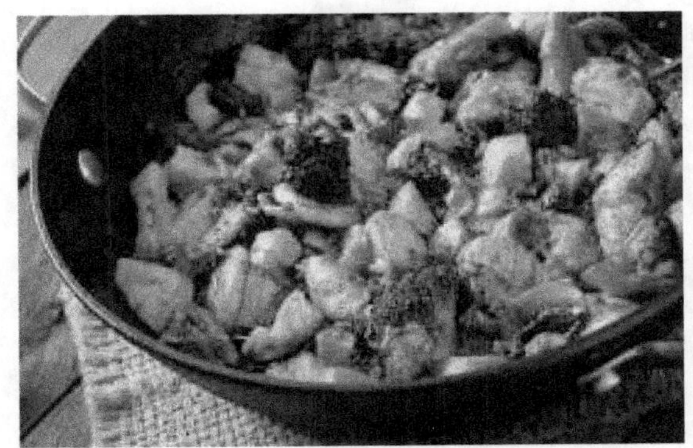

Preparation Time: 15 minutes

Cooking Time: 25 minutes

Servings: 6

Ingredients:

3 tablespoons olive oil

1 pound skinless, boneless chicken breast, cubed

1 medium onion, chopped - 6 garlic cloves, minced

2 cups fresh mushrooms, sliced - 16 ounces small broccoli florets

¼ cup water

Salt and ground black pepper, to taste

Directions:

Heat the oil in a large saucepan over medium heat and cook the chicken cubes for about 4–5 minutes.

With a slotted spoon, transfer the chicken cubes onto a plate.

In the same wok, add the onion and sauté for about 4–5 minutes.

Add the mushrooms and cook for about 4–5 minutes. Stir in the cooked chicken, broccoli, and water, and cook (covered) for about 8–10 minutes, stirring occasionally. Stir in salt and black pepper and remove from heat. Serve hot.

Nutrition:

Calories 197 Fat 10.1 g Carbs 8.5 g   Protein 20.1 g

CHAPTER 15:

Snack Recipes

Rosemary Toasted Walnuts

Preparation Time: 10 minutes

Cooking Time: 20 minutes

Servings: 8

Ingredients:

2 cups raw walnuts

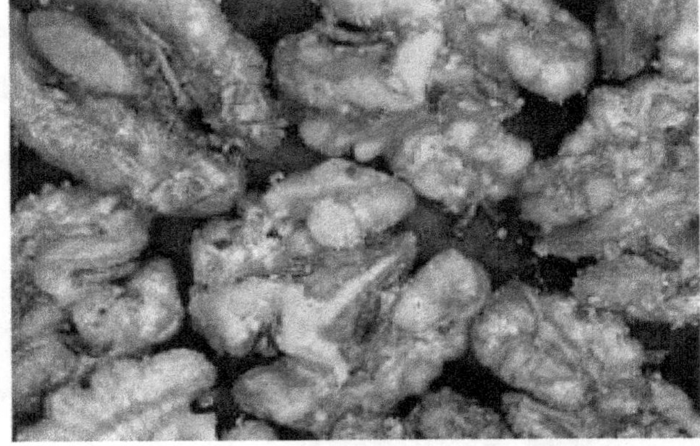

2 tablespoons fresh rosemary, finely chopped - ¼ cup olive oil - ½ teaspoon salt - 1 teaspoon pepper

Directions:

Preheat oven to 350° F. Line a baking sheet with parchment paper.

In a bowl, whisk together olive oil, rosemary, salt, and pepper.

Add in walnuts and toss until completely covered in olive oil mixture.

Bake the walnuts for 10-15 minutes in the oven, tossing every 4-5 minutes until they're golden brown. The walnuts cook quickly, so be careful not to burn them. Enjoy!

Nutrition:

Calories 223 Fat 23g Carbohydrates 5g Protein 4g

Dark Chocolate Pretzel Cookies

Preparation Time: 20 minutes

Cooking Time: 15 minutes

Servings: 3

Ingredients:

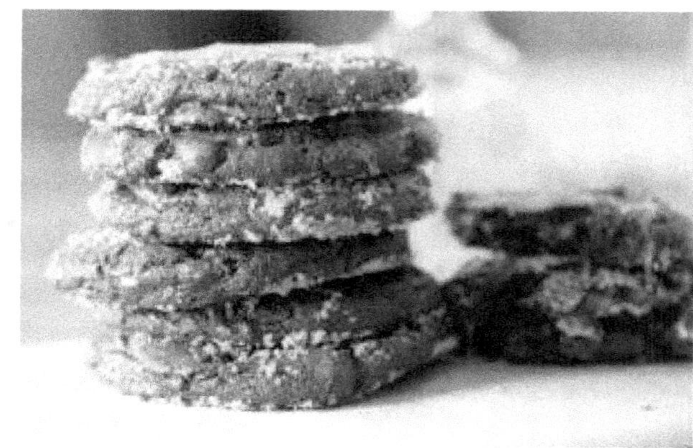

1 cup yogurt - 1/2 tsp baking soda

1/4 teaspoon salt - 1/4 tsp cinnamon - 4 tbsp. butter softened - 1/3 cup brown sugar

1 egg - 1/2 tsp vanilla - 1/2 cup dark chocolate chips

1/2 cup pretzels chopped

Directions:

Preheat oven to 350 degrees.

At a medium bowl, whisk together the sugar, butter, vanilla, and egg.

In another bowl, stir together the flour, baking soda, and salt.

Stir the bread mixture in using all the moist components, along with the chocolate chips and pretzels until just blended.

Drop large spoonful of dough on an unlined baking sheet.

Bake it for 15-17 minutes or until the bottoms are somewhat all crispy.

Allow cooling on a wire rack.

Nutrition:

Calories 130 Fat 7g Carbohydrates 19g Protein 3g

Strawberry Buckwheat Tabbouleh

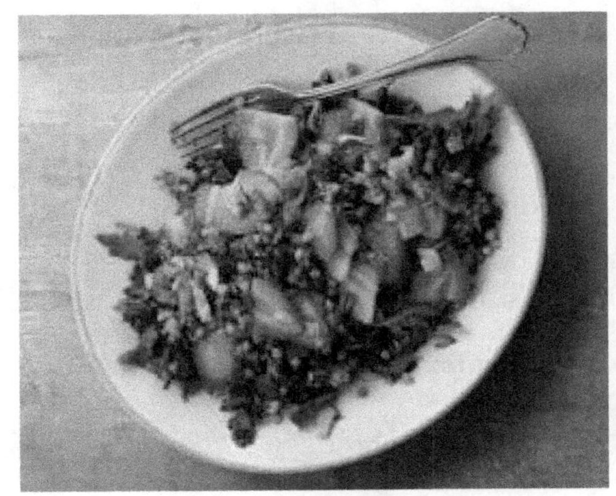

Preparation Time: 5 minutes

Cooking Time: 5 minutes

Servings: 3

Ingredients:

50 g buckwheat - 1 tbsp. ground turmeric

80 g avocado - 65 g tomato - 20 g red onion

25 g Medjool dates, pitted - 1 tbsp. capers - 30 g parsley - 100 g strawberries, hulled

1 tbsp. extra virgin olive oil

Juice from 1/2 lemon

30 g rocket

Directions:

Cook the buckwheat with the turmeric as guided by the package. Drain to cool and keep to one side.

Chop the tomato, avocado, dates, red onion, capers, and parsley thinly.

Mix them with the cool buckwheat.

Slice the strawberries, and mix the oil and lemon juice gently into the salad. Serve up on a rocket bed.

Nutrition:

Calories 226 Fat 8.3g

Carbohydrates 23.7g Protein 12.4g

Artichoke with Three Cheeses

Preparation Time: 20 minutes

Cooking Time: 40 minutes

Servings: 4

Ingredients:

2 cups artichoke hearts

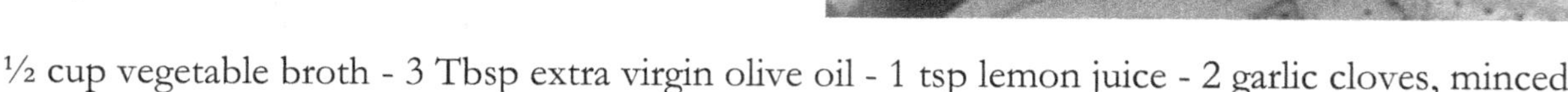

½ cup vegetable broth - 3 Tbsp extra virgin olive oil - 1 tsp lemon juice - 2 garlic cloves, minced

Fresh parsley, chopped - Fresh basil, chopped

½ cup shredded Fontina cheese

½ cup of shredded Swiss cheese

½ cup shredded Parmesan cheese

Directions:

Preheat oven to 400F

Arrange artichokes in single layer of a deep baking dish. Drizzle oil, lemon juice, garlic, vegetable broth over the artichokes. Start with fontina cheese, then Swiss cheese, parmesan cheese last.

Cover baking dish with aluminum foil. Bake 15 minutes.

Remove foil. Bake an additional 15 minutes, until cheese is golden and bubbly.

Remove from oven. Let it cool to room temperature. Serve.

Nutrition:

Calories: 57 Fat: 14g Carbs: 3g Protein: 4g Dietary Fiber: 2.6g

Raw Vegan Coffee Cashew Cream Cake

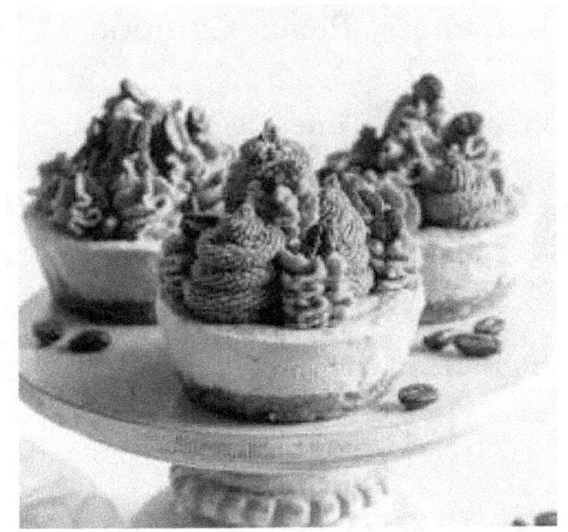

Preparation Time: 10 minutes

Cooking Time: 35 minutes

Servings: 4

Ingredients:

Coffee cashew cream

2 cups raw cashews

1 tsp of ground vanilla bean

3 tbsp. melted coconut oil

¼ cup raw honey

1/3 cup very strong coffee or triple espresso shot

For the crust:

See recipe for Raw Walnuts Pie Crust

Directions:

Blend all ingredients for the cream, pour it onto the crust and refrigerate.

Garnish with coffee beans.

Nutrition:

Calories 153

Carbs 22g

Fat 1g Protein 2g

Blackberry Peach Compote

Preparation Time: 10 minutes

Cooking Time: 20 minutes

Servings: 12

Ingredients:

¼ cup Sauvignon Blanc wine

2 Tbsps. Xylitol

1 tsp ground ginger

1 tsp Cinnamon

3 medium peaches

¼ cup blackberries

½ tsp thick it up

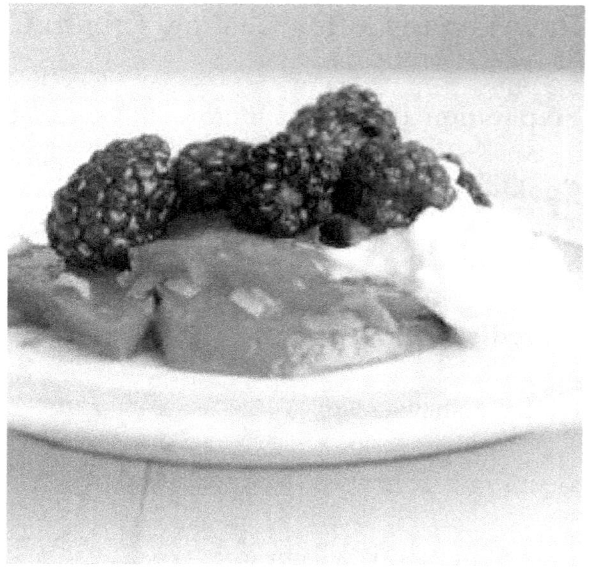

Directions:

In a large saucepan, combine the wine, Xylitol, ginger, peaches, and cinnamon.

Simmer for 15 minutes.

Add the blackberries. Simmer another 5 minutes, until berries are tender.

Stir in the thick it up. Simmer approximately 5 minutes.

Remove from heat. Cool to room temperature. Serve.

Nutrition:

Calories: 35 Fat: 0.2g Carbs: 4.2g Protein: 0.5g Dietary Fiber: 3.4g

CHAPTER 16:

Dinner Recipes

Chicken Breast with Asparagus

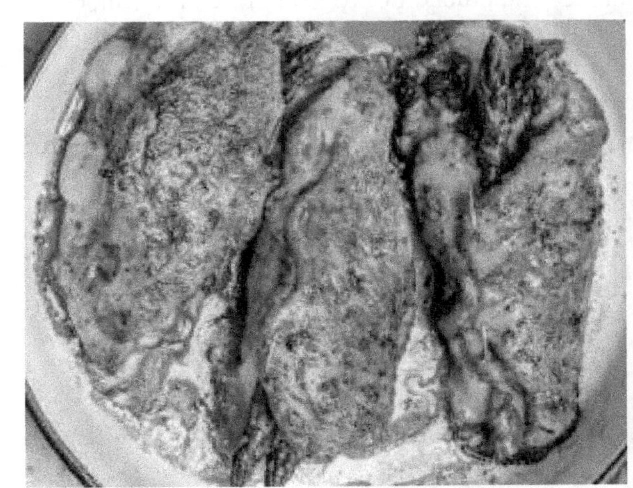

Preparation Time: 15 minutes

Cooking Time: 16 minutes

Servings: 5

Ingredients:

For Chicken:

¼ cup extra-virgin olive oil

¼ cup fresh lemon juice - 2 tablespoons maple syrup - 1 garlic clove, minced

Salt and ground black pepper, as required - 5 (6-ounce) boneless, skinless chicken breasts

For Asparagus:

1½ pounds fresh asparagus - 2 tablespoons extra-virgin olive oil - 1 tablespoon fresh lemon juice

Directions:

For marinade: in a large bowl, add oil, lemon juice, Erythritol, garlic, salt and black pepper and beat until well combined.

In a large resealable plastic bag, place the chicken and ¾ cup of marinade.

Seal the bag and shake to coat well.

Refrigerate overnight.

Cover the bowl of remaining marinade and refrigerate before serving.

Preheat the grill to medium heat. Grease the grill grate.

Remove the chicken from bag and discard the marinade.

Place the chicken onto grill grate and grill, covered for about 5-8 minutes per side.

Meanwhile, in a pan of boiling water, arrange a steamer basket.

Place the asparagus in steamer basket and steam, covered for about 5-7 minutes.

Drain the asparagus well and transfer into a bowl.

Add oil and lemon juice and toss to coat well.

Divide the chicken breasts and asparagus onto serving plates and serve.

Nutrition:

Calories: 520

Fat: 29.7g

Cholesterol: 151mg

Sodium: 184mg

Carbohydrates: 11.2g

Fiber: 2.9g

Sugar: 7.7g

Protein: 52.4g

Beef with Kale & Carrot

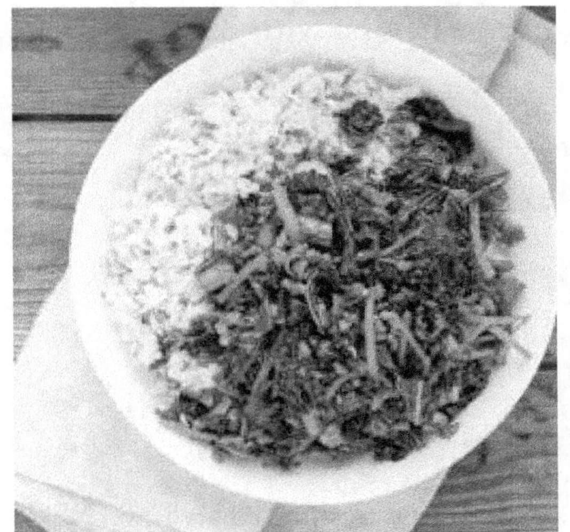

Preparation Time: 15 minutes

Cooking Time: 12 minutes

Servings: 4

Ingredients:

2 tablespoons coconut oil

4 garlic cloves, minced

1 pound beef sirloin steak, cut into bite-sized pieces

Ground black pepper, as required

1½ cups carrots, peeled and cut into matchsticks

1½ cups fresh kale, tough ribs removed and chopped

3 tablespoons low-sodium soy sauce

Directions:

Melt the coconut oil in a wok over medium heat and sauté the garlic for about 1 minute.

Add the beef and black pepper and stir to combine. Increase the heat to medium-high and cook for about 3-4 minutes or until browned from all sides. Add the carrot, kale and tamari and cook for about 4-5 minutes. Remove from the heat and serve hot.

Nutrition:

Calories: 311 Fat: 13.8g Cholesterol: 101mg Sodium: 700mg Carbohydrates: 8.4g

Fiber: 1.6g Sugar: 2.3g Protein: 37.1g

Lamb Chops with Kale

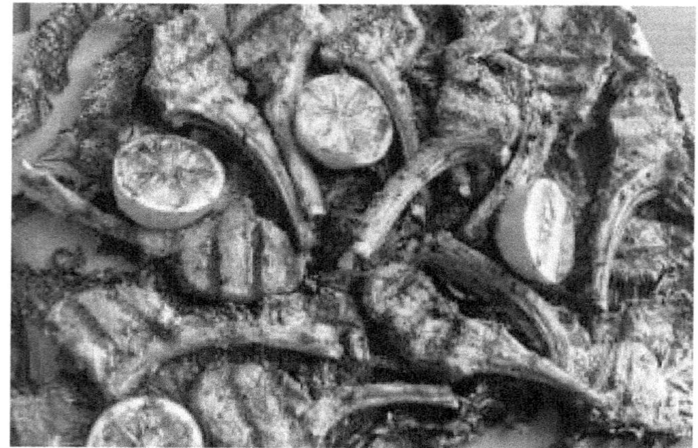

Preparation Time: 15 minutes

Cooking Time: 11 minutes

Servings: 4

Ingredients:

1 garlic clove, minced

1 tablespoon fresh rosemary leaves, minced

Salt and ground black pepper, as required

4 lamb loin chops

4 cups fresh baby kale

Directions:

Preheat the grill to high heat. Grease the grill grate.

In a bowl, add the garlic, rosemary, salt and black pepper and mix well.

Coat the lamb chops with the herb mixture generously.

Place the chops onto the hot side of grill and cook for about 2 minutes per side.

Now, move the chops onto the cooler side of the grill and cook for about 6-7 minutes.

Divide the kale onto serving plates and top each with 1 chop. Serve immediately.

Nutrition:

Calories: 301 Fat: 10.5g Cholesterol: 128mg Sodium: 176mg Carbohydrates: 7.8g Fiber: 1.4g

Sugar: 0g Protein: 41.9g

Salmon with Arugula

Preparation Time: 15 minutes

Cooking Time: 8 minutes

Servings: 4

Ingredients:

For Salmon:

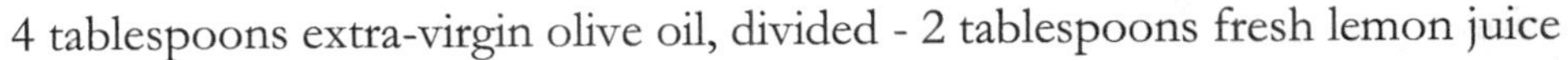

4 tablespoons extra-virgin olive oil, divided - 2 tablespoons fresh lemon juice

1 teaspoon ground turmeric - 1 teaspoon ground cumin - Salt and ground black pepper, as required

4 (4-ounce) boneless, skinless salmon fillets

For Salad:

6 cups fresh arugula - 2 cups cherry tomatoes, halved

Directions:

In a bowl, mix together 2 tablespoons of oil, lemon juice, turmeric, cumin, salt and black pepper.

Add the salmon fillets and coat with the oil mixture generously. Set aside.

In a non-stick wok, heat remaining oil over medium heat. Place salmon fillets, skin-side down and cook for about 3-5 minutes.

Change the side and cook for about 2-3 minutes more. Divide the salmon, arugula and tomatoes onto serving plates and serve immediately.

Nutrition:

Calories: 299 Fat: 21.6g Cholesterol: 50mg Sodium: 104mg Carbohydrates: 5.4g

Fiber: 1.8g Sugar: 3.2g Protein: 23.8g

Chickpeas with Swiss Chard

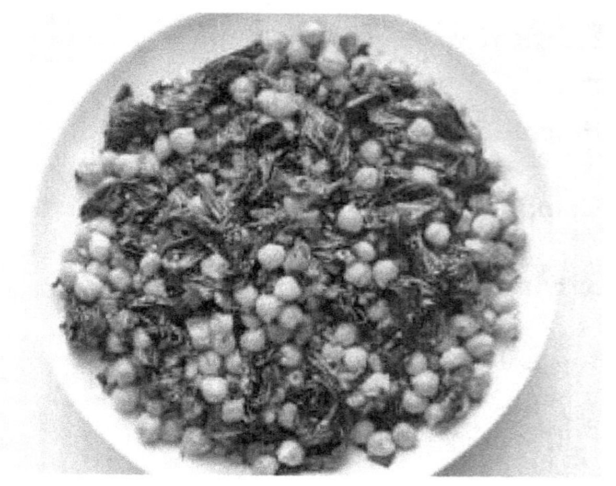

Preparation Time: 15 minutes

Cooking Time: 12 minutes

Servings: 4

Ingredients:

2 tablespoon extra-virgin olive oil

2 garlic cloves, sliced thinly

1 large tomato, chopped finely - 2 bunches fresh Swiss chard, trimmed

1 (18-ounce) can chickpeas, drained and rinsed - Salt and ground black pepper, as required

¼ cup water - 1 tablespoon fresh lemon juice

2 tablespoons fresh parsley, chopped

Directions:

Heat the oil in a large wok over medium heat and sauté the garlic for about 1 minute.

Add the tomato and cook for about 2-3 minutes, crushing with the back of spoon.

Stir in remaining ingredients except lemon juice and parsley and cook for about 5-7 minutes.

Drizzle with the lemon juice and remove from the heat.

Serve hot with the garnishing of parsley.

Nutrition:

Calories: 217 Fat: 8.3g Cholesterol: 0mg Sodium: 171mg Carbohydrates: 26.2g

Fiber: 6g Sugar: 1.8g Protein: 8.8g

Buckwheat Noodles with Chicken

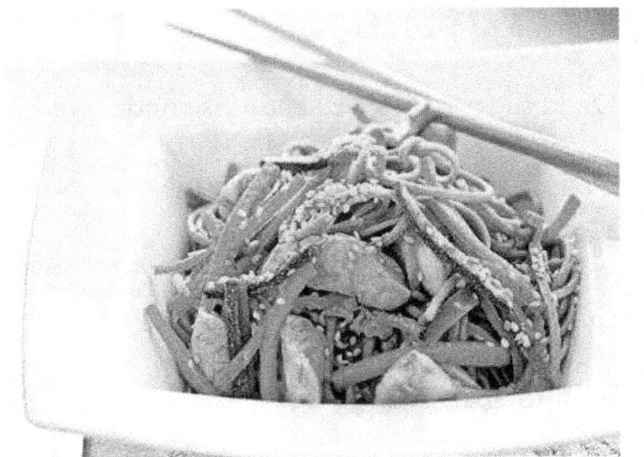

Preparation Time: 20 minutes

Cooking Time: 17 minutes

Servings: 4

Ingredients:

1 pound boneless chicken tenderloins

Salt and ground black pepper, as required

8 ounces buckwheat noodles

3 tablespoons extra-virgin olive oil, divided

6 garlic cloves, chopped finely

8 ounces fresh mushrooms, sliced thinly

1 cup carrots, peeled and julienned

¼ cup low-sodium soy sauce

3 tablespoons red wine vinegar

1 tablespoon maple syrup

1 tablespoon sesame seeds

Directions:

Arrange the chicken tenderloins between 2 sheets of plastic wrap and wit a meat mallet, pound slightly to flatten.

Season the chicken tenderloins with salt and black pepper lightly and set aside.

In a pan of the lightly salted boiling water, cook the buckwheat noodles for about 5 minutes.

Drain the noodles well and rinse under cold water.

Drain the noodles again and set aside.

In a large non-stick wok, heat 2 tablespoons of the olive oil over medium-high heat and cook the chicken tenders for about 2 minutes per side.

With tongs, place the chicken tenders onto a cutting board to allow cool.

Cut the chicken tenderloins into ¼-inch pieces diagonally.

In the same wok, heat the remaining olive oil over medium heat and sauté the garlic for about 1 minute.

Add the mushrooms and stir-fry for about 5 minutes longer.

Add the carrot and stir-fry for about 2 minutes.

Remove the wok from the heat and stir in chicken pieces.

In a small bowl, add soy sauce, vinegar and maple syrup and beat until well combined.

In a large serving bowl, add noodles, chicken mixture and sauce mixture and toss to coat well.

Serve immediately.

Nutrition:

Calories: 447 Fat: 13.3g

Cholesterol: 71mg Sodium: 1500mg

Carbohydrates: 4g.7 Fiber: 3g

Sugar: 6.4g Protein: 33.1g

CHAPTER 17:

Dessert Recipes

Chocolate Mousse

Preparation Time: 6 mins

Cooking Time: 0 mins

Servings: 6

Ingredients:

16 ounces (2 cups) cream cheese - 3-6 tablespoons of the desired sweetener

1/2 cup unsweetened cocoa powder - 1/2 cup heavy whipped cream - One large avocado

90% dark chocolate, to garnish - 1/4 teaspoon vanilla extract

Directions:

Beat cream cheese until it becomes smooth and creamy, slowly mix cocoa powder. Add avocado and beat it nicely for 5 minutes until it becomes creamy. Add vanilla and sweetener, and then hit it again until it becomes creamy and smooth.

Place the whipped cream in the chocolate mixture and fold gently. Place the chocolate mousse in the desired containers. Garnish with dark chocolate chips.

Nutrition:

Calories: 333 Cal Fat: 35 g Fiber: g Carbs: 2 g Protein: 1 g

Chocolate Chia Pudding with Almonds

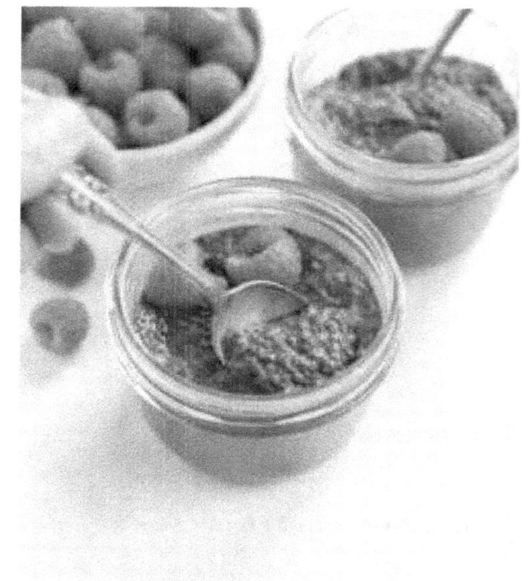

Preparation Time: 10 mins

Cooking Time: 0 mins

Servings: 2

Ingredients:

4 tablespoons of chopped almonds

1 cup of water

Sweetener

½ cup heavy cream

2 tablespoons of cocoa powder

6 tablespoons of chia seeds

2 tablespoons of MCT oil

Directions:

Add chia seeds, heavy cream, water, MCT oil, cocoa powder, and sweetener in a bowl.

Mix them. Allow sitting for 7-11 hours. After 11 hours, add almonds. Your dish is ready.

Nutrition:

Calories: 288 Cal

Fat: 28 g Fiber: 8 g

Carbs: 3 g Protein: 4 g

Coconut Macadamia Chia Pudding

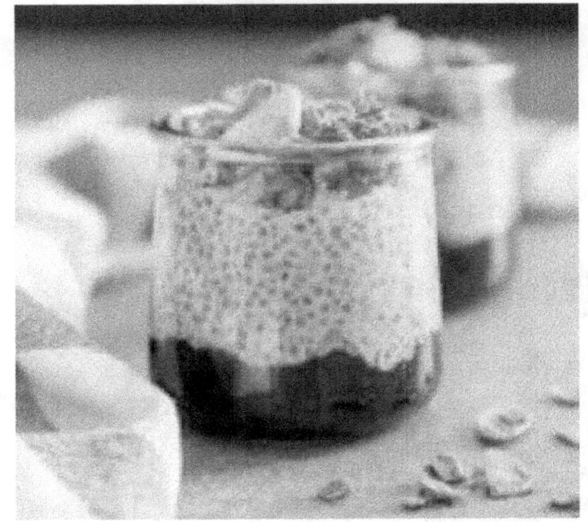

Preparation Time: 10 mins

Cooking Time: 0 mins

Servings: 3

Ingredients:

4 tablespoons of macadamia nuts (chopped)

1 cup of water

Sweetener

½ cup coconut cream

2 tablespoons of MCT oil

6 tablespoons of chia seeds

Directions:

Add chia seeds, coconut cream, water, MCT oil and sweetener in a bowl. Mix them.

Allow sitting for 7-11 hours.

After 11 hours add macadamia nuts. Your dish is ready.

Nutrition:

Calories: 260 Cal

Fat: 9 g Fiber: 2 g

Carbs: 2 g Protein: 2 g

Chocolate Mug

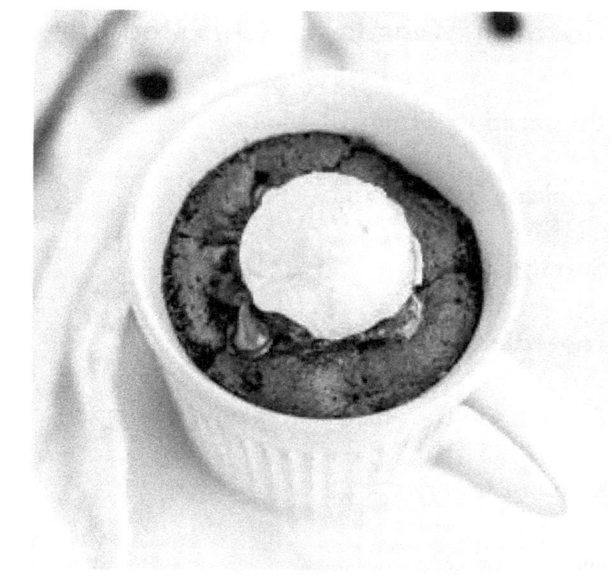

Preparation Time: 7 mins

Cooking Time: 0 mins

Servings: 1

Ingredients:

2 tablespoons of butter

1 teaspoon sweetener

1/4 cup almond powder

1/2 teaspoon baking powder

Two tablespoons of cocoa powder

Pinch of salt

1 big beaten egg

1/4 cup whipped cream, to serve

2 tablespoons of Keto-based chocolate chips

Directions:

Place the butter in a microwaveable cup and heat until melted for 30 seconds.

Add remaining ingredients except for whipped cream and stir well.

Microwave for 45 seconds to 1 minute, or until the cake set, but still fudgy. Serve with cream.

Nutrition:

Calories: 500 Cal Fat: 50 g Fiber: 3 g Carbs: 2 g Protein: 7 g

Vanilla Chia Pudding

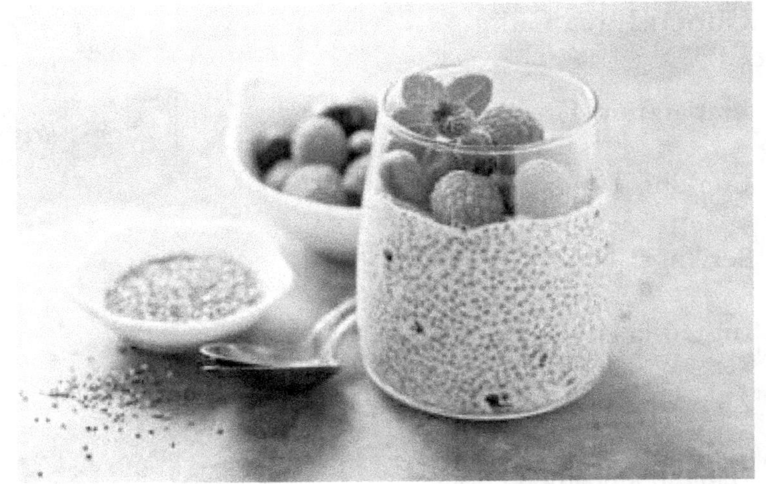

Preparation Time: 5 mins

Cooking Time: 0 mins

Servings: 1

Ingredients:

1/2 cup strawberries

2 cups of water

Sweetener

½ cup heavy cream

Vanilla extract (few drops)

½ cup chia seeds

2 tablespoons MCT oil

Directions:

Add chia seeds, heavy cream, water, MCT oil, vanilla extract, and sweetener in a bowl.

Mix them. Allow sitting for 7-11 hours.

After 11 hours, add strawberries. Your dish is ready.

Nutrition:

Calories: 550 Cal Fat: 57 g

Fiber: 3 g Carbs: 12 g

Protein: 2 g

Choco Lava Cake

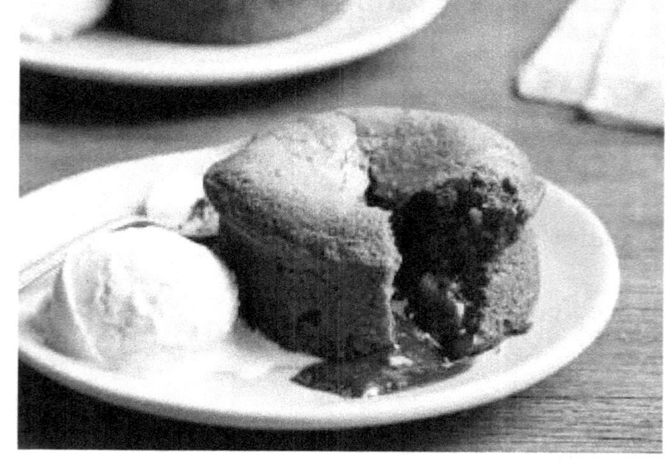

Preparation Time: 20 mins

Cooking Time: 0 mins

Servings: 4

Ingredients:

2.5 ounces of dark chocolate

1tablespoon almond flour

1/4 cup coconut oil - 1/4 teaspoon Vanilla extract - 2 eggs - Cocoa powder for garnish

2 tablespoons of sweetener

Directions:

Preheat oven to 375 ° C.

Grease two molds with coconut oil and sprinkle them with cocoa powder.

Melt chocolate, coconut oil and add vanilla to it.

Beat eggs and sweetener together in a different bowl.

Slowly add the chocolate mixture with egg mixture and beat until well mixed.

Add the almond flour and mix until incorporated.

Fill the molds evenly with the dough.

Bake for 10 minutes. Serve immediately.

Nutrition:

Calories: 247 Cal Fat: 24 g Fiber: 0 g Carbs: 2 g Protein: 3 g

Conclusion

There are a thousand and one different diets to lose weight. Every day, a new method to lose weight appears that leaves us homiletics, and that makes us jump on the bandwagon of diets that promise results in a very short time.

Although not all of these diets are healthy, there are some that have risen to fame due to the celebrities who have followed it. The last to jump into the fray?

The sirtfood diet that promises to make you lose around three kilos a week, and that seems, Adele has followed to lose 70 kilos.

While half the world is waiting for Adele to release a new album, the other half is obsessed with her weight change. And the rumors are that he would have succeeded with the Sirtfood diet.

This diet began to be a trend since it included the option of including dark chocolate and wine to the nutritional plan. The Sirtfood diet is quite simple and easy to get around since it focuses on foods get from sources of a plant. It encourages fruit, vegetables, whole grains, legumes, seeds, and nuts to eat, which means that most of what you eat is made up of these foods.

You may think it's a vegetarian diet or classic vegan at first. It is not just a diet based on plants; it is flexible considerably and does not boycott milk, seafood, meat, and eggs. It's easy-going and inclusive approach makes this diet attractive–after all, no one likes rules!

Sirtfood also helps preserve muscles, the tissue with the highest energy consumption. Sit-ins activate muscle stem cells. This works on the same principle as strength training: muscles are stressed - here by exertion, in the diet by lack of energy - the repair mechanism starts, new muscle mass is created. More muscle means more energy consumption and is the best remedy for the yo-yo effect.

The Sirtfood Diet is a diet of addition, not isolation, and Sirtfoods are widely accessible and affordable for all. This is a diet that can help you lose weight and boost your metabolism.

You have not only learned the basic information required to start the Sirtfood diet, but you have also gained much more than that! By learning how to meal plan, prep, and storage, you will be able to easily master the Sirt food diet with little day-to-day effort required.

You will be able to enjoy delicious meals at a moment's notice without having to struggle after a long day of work. By just preparing a little ahead of time, you can have a fridge and freezer fully stocked with delicious homemade meals perfectly suited to your taste.

Whether you start out following the Sirt diet to the letter or simply experimenting and enjoying the dishes, you are sure to experience benefits and fall in love with food all over again.

What are you waiting for? With just a little effort and time in the kitchen, you can get on your way to success.

Always remember that feeling good about your body is the key to many achievements. It helps you become more confident to do lots of things. Your life has a great value, you should be able to maximize what it has to offer.